the weekend-off diet

Diet Monday to Friday and lose weight

Helen Foster

hamlyn

First published in Great Britain in 2006 by
Hamlyn, an imprint of Octopus Publishing Group Ltd
2–4 Heron Quays, London E14 4JP

ISBN-13: 978-0-600-61246-9

ISBN-10: 0-600-61246-5

A CIP catalogue record for this book is available from the British
Library

Printed and bound in Spain

10 9 8 7 6 5 4 3 2 1

It is advisable to check with your doctor before embarking on any
exercise or diet plan. The advice given in this book should not be
considered a replacement for professional medical treatment. While
the information given here is believed to be accurate and the step-by-
step instructions have been devised to avoid strain, neither the author
nor the publisher can accept any legal responsibility for any injury or
illness sustained while following the exercises and diet plan.

contents

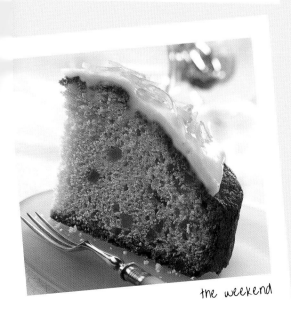

the diet week

the exercise week

the weekend

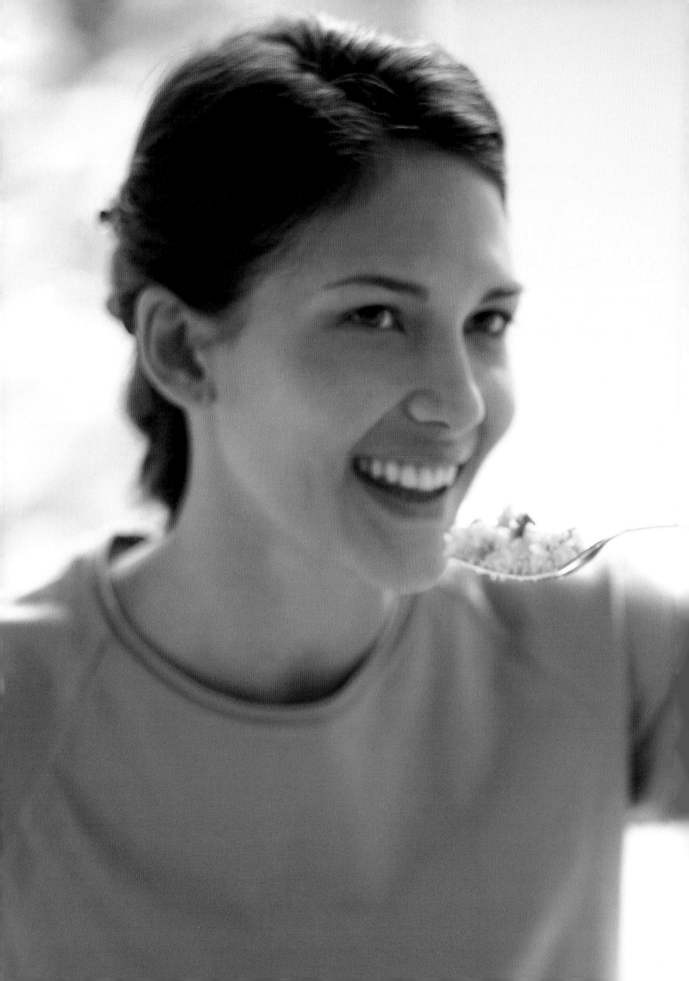

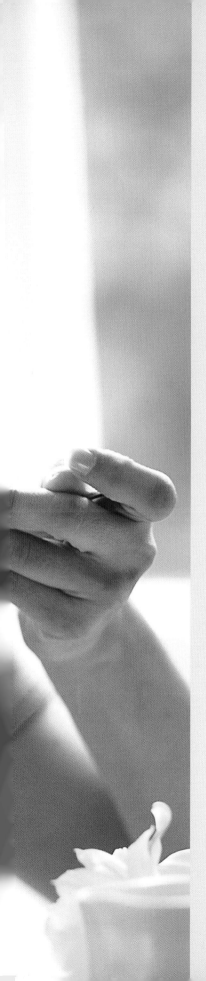

introduction

Welcome to the easiest diet you've ever thought
about starting. If you tend to associate diets with
deprivation, endless longings for favourite foods
and hunger pangs that stalk you day and night,
then it's time for you to think again about what it
takes to lose weight. Science now reveals that the
starvation approach normal diets tend to take
actually works against your body's natural weight-
loss mechanisms, making it harder than it need
be to lose weight. You don't need to be hungry to
be slim and you don't need to give up your
favourite foods either – and we're about to prove
this in the pages that follow. Keep reading and
we'll tell you everything you need to know to get
in the best shape of your life.

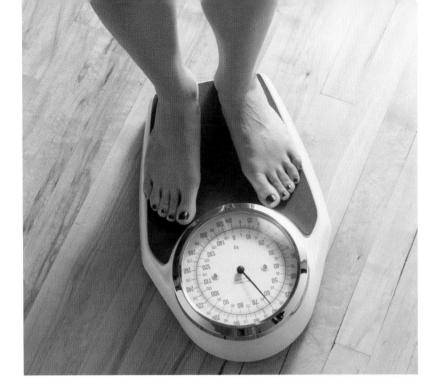

Introducing the diet

If the phrase 'I'll start my diet again on Monday' means anything to you, then you've just picked up the right book. A reader survey carried out by a popular health magazine revealed that the average dieter will go on 32 diets in their lifetime, and will last an average of 42 days on each one before giving up. And that's the strict dieters.

Perpetual dieting

A 2004 study from UK retailer Marks & Spencer found that 50 per cent of female dieters and 40 per cent of male ones quit within the first four weeks of their plan. The reason for this is very familiar to most of us. We get to Friday night, enjoy a few drinks or a meal out, go over our allotted calorie/carbohydrate/fat allowance and think, 'Well that's that then. I might as well give up this weekend and start again on Monday.' The result is that you always seem to be on a diet, but the weight never actually comes off.

You want to be a thin person – not a different one

Most traditional diets fail for one very good reason. They forget that people who gain weight tend to do so because they like eating – food isn't just something eaten to stop fainting, it's something that has enjoyment attached to it. Going on a diet that bans treats and makes eating out either impossible or guilt wracked therefore doesn't just mean changing your eating habits, it means changing who you are and what you enjoy. As a result it's a chore, and it's also pretty much guaranteed to fail on the first day that the needle on the scales doesn't move.

Furthermore, if you weren't that bothered about food before you went on your diet, you will be once things get under way. According to a survey commissioned by Sveltesse Cereal Bars, 66 per cent of people report that as soon as they go on a diet they start craving the foods they're not supposed to eat more intensely than normal and their intake actually goes up. Even more worrying, US scientist Ancel Keys conducted studies of army recruits put on diets and showed that it took just days before they became so

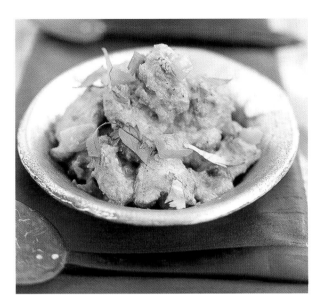

a deep pan pizza every day yet still lose weight. Sadly, that just cannot happen. On this diet, like most others, you'll be eating high levels of fruit and vegetables, you'll swap full-fat milk for skimmed, and low-fat snacks will replace some of the chocolate, potato crisps and cakes you currently eat. What makes this diet different, however, is that these food swaps don't happen every single day. Remember, it's called the 'Weekend-off Diet', and that's exactly what you do. You take the weekend off from dieting and so wave goodbye to the feelings of deprivation normally associated with losing weight.

What it all means

It means you end up with a diet plan you can stick with long enough to get results, whether you're aiming for a weight loss of 3 kg (7 lb) or 30 kg (66 lb). But, more importantly, it means you also regain a sense of control around food. You are never going to live a life where you don't encounter fatty or sugary foods so why should you diet as if that is the case. From day one on this plan, not only do you learn how to eat to lose weight, but you learn tactics that help you control yourself around food. When you've finished this plan, those traditionally forbidden foods should have no adverse effect on your waistline. In other words, this is the diet plan that will finally teach you to eat happily for life.

fixated with food that they started collecting recipes and thinking about careers as chefs. It's clear that banning treats completely on a diet doesn't work – yet diet plan after diet plan depends on you doing that. The Weekend-off Diet, however, does not.

Feel healthy not hungry

On this diet plan treats and favourite foods are encouraged rather than banned. That's not to say that this diet allows you to eat packets of biscuits or

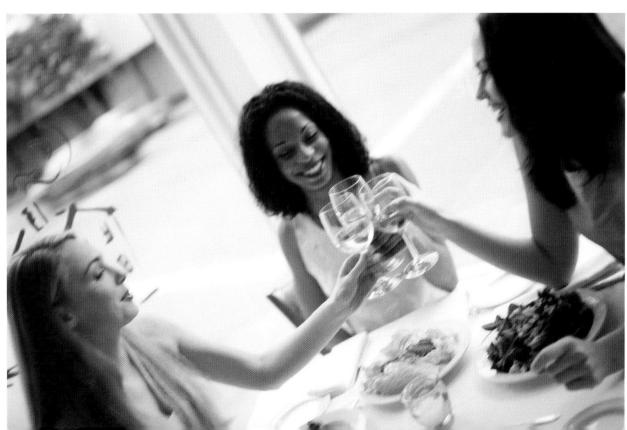

What does the diet involve?

This diet really is simple. For five days a week you follow a structured low-calorie, nutrient-rich, metabolism-boosting diet and exercise plan. Then for the two days of the weekend you can eat whatever you like. Essentially, you divide your dieting life, just as most of us divide our weeks – into weekdays and weekend days with different rules for each.

Weekdays

Whatever diet they are on, most dieters find it fairly easy to stick to their diet plan during the week. There's lots of reasons for this – you're usually too busy to cheat, if you're at work or out and about there's no easily available fridge or cupboard of goodies to tempt you, and you probably have less of a social life during the week to derail things. The result is that weekdays are definitely more diet friendly and it's the reason why, on this diet, you're going to stick to an organized eating plan from Monday to Friday.

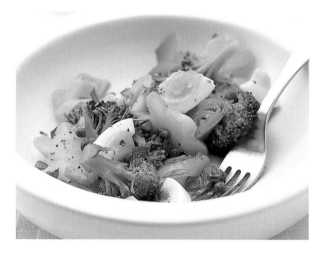

This plan contains three low-calorie but high-nutrient meals a day, plus a couple of snacks. It's full of foods that fill you up, but it's also planned around high levels of foods shown to boost your metabolism and encourage fat burning, which potentially increases your weight loss further, instead of eating the same number of calories made up from other foods. This combination calorie boost means that it is Monday to Friday when you'll primarily lose weight on this diet plan. Over the weekend all you're aiming to do is maintain your weight loss, ready to start the next diet spurt again come Monday.

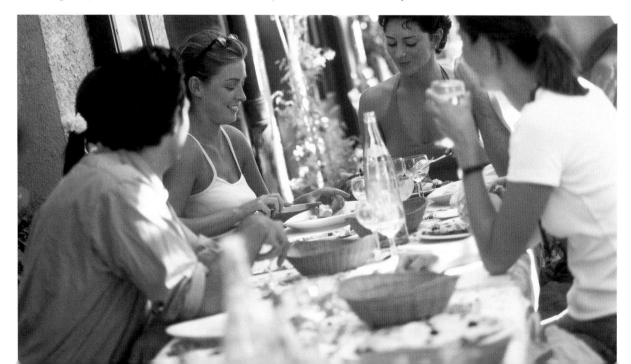

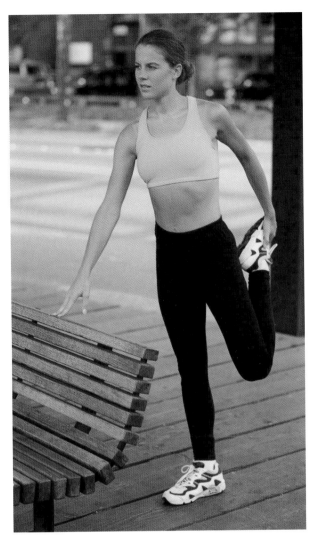

triggering the associated guilt binge. As every hour of your weekend off ticks by, your motivation renews so that by the time Monday comes you'll be ready to repeat your successes of the week before. It might sound like a gimmick but there are actually good scientific reasons why this diet can work.

The role of exercise

Exercise is a vital part of any weight loss plan. It burns calories while you do it and creates a metabolic boost that means you continue burning calories at a higher rate when you stop exercising (see page 22). On this diet you'll be doing three types of exercise:

- During the week you'll be doing 'stealth exercise', which you'll build into your day potentially without even noticing.

- In addition, you'll do a simple 8- to 10-minute daily toning plan to help rev up your metabolism and firm up your muscles from top to toe.

- At weekends you'll do a little more activity as you'll need to balance out your extra food intake, but it'll be something that you choose to do and that you really enjoy.

At the moment you might see exercise – like most diets – as a chore, but when you realize that exercise doesn't need to involve the gym, nor pain and discomfort, and in some cases not even need a tracksuit and trainers, you'll realize that exercising can brighten up and energize your weekend, as well as power up your weight loss.

Don't be afraid of the exercise part of the plan. Aim to enjoy it and you might find that you change more about your life than just your weight over the next few weeks or months. After all, taking part in a regular exercise programme has been shown to improve your energy levels and mood, to help maximize your immunity, to promote deeper, sounder sleep and even help to boost your sex life – not to mention the fact that with every step you take you are reducing your risk of serious, long-term illnesses like heart disease and cancer. It really is an all-round way to makeover your body.

Weekends

At weekends you'll relax a bit – just like you do mentally and physically when the usual Monday to Friday routine stops. From Saturday morning until Sunday night you can eat any food you like – chocolate, chips, Chinese takeouts, anything you like – just as long as you stick to some simple guidelines (see The Weekend, page 102). In a nutshell, these guidelines teach you to get back in touch with your body so you can determine what it really needs in terms of the food you eat. Taking time off dieting every weekend also means you'll effectively recharge your diet batteries. You'll be able to give in to any cravings you've had during the week so they won't plague you next week and stall your weight loss, and you can enjoy social events without feeling that you're cheating and

Why the diet works

Having a break from dieting on Saturday and Sunday may seem too good to be true, but there are some sound reasons for the success of this plan. These include no more feelings of guilt, deprivation or boredom; your metabolism is maintained and you learn to control yourself around fattening foods.

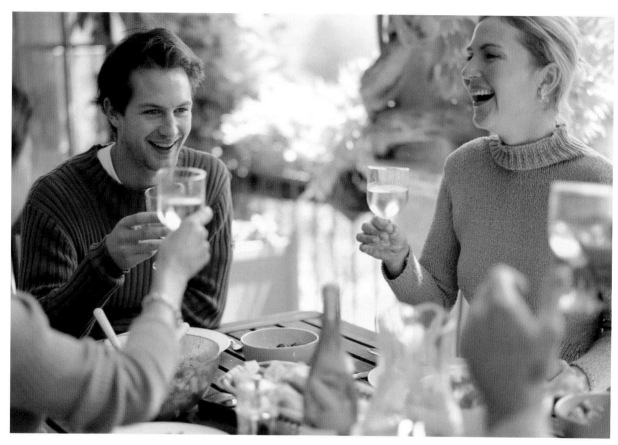

It's the guilt-free diet

Weekends are generally the most destructive time for diets: we have less of a routine to keep us focused, food is more readily available and many of us like to socialize over a good meal.

In calorie terms, the extra food we normally eat over the weekend isn't actually that bad – studies conducted by the US University of North Carolina School of Public Health showed that we take in only 115 calories more a day – but when we're dieting many of us develop an 'all or nothing' mentality. If we break our diet, even by one biscuit, we tend to

think 'that's that' and then we binge. This leads to overeating for the rest of the day and often continues with an increased amount of consumption until the Monday morning, when we feel psychologically ready to start again on our current diet attempt. The result is that when we're dieting, our increased weekend intake can end up far higher than those 115 extra calories we'd have eaten normally. On this diet, this doesn't happen. We can eat what we want at weekends and know we're not breaking our diet, so there's no guilt – and, above all, we're much less likely to binge.

It keeps your metabolism up

Our bodies are designed for survival and don't know when we're trying to lose weight. If you cut calories too low for more than four or five days your body thinks food has suddenly become scarce. As a result, it prepares itself to survive on fewer calories by slowing your metabolism and reducing the amount of fat it releases from its fat stores. Not surprisingly, this slows your weight loss as well.

This diet prevents this in two ways. Firstly, during the week you're eating regularly, which naturally raises metabolism. In addition, you're supplying your body with high levels of nutrients and metabolism-boostingfoods, both of which also keep things revved up. Secondly, when the weekend comes and the body receives a calorific increase, it no longer thinks food is scarce and it doesn't go into that conservation mode.

You don't get bored

As recent research from the UK revealed (see page 6), the average person sticks to a traditional diet plan for just four weeks. This is because they get bored of restricting their diet to certain foods and miss their favourite treats. If you have only a little weight to lose this short time span is no problem, but for long-term weight loss, it can lead to heartache and frustration as you stop and start various diets, never finding one that fits your likes or lifestyle. On this diet, however, since you follow a diet plan for only five days at a time before you can treat yourself, staying motivated is much easier.

You're less likely to eat 'invisible' calories

The longer you're on a normal diet, the more likely it is that invisible calories creep in. They come from stopping weighing portions because you think you know how much is right, or because weight loss is going so well that you figure the odd chocolate bar won't hurt. Eventually the calories add up. Because this diet effectively lasts only five days each time (and in between you can have your potato crisps or cheese or chocolate), it's much easier to avoid these invisible calories.

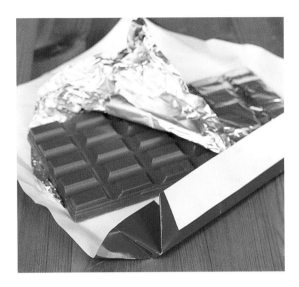

Why crash dieting doesn't work

The slowdown in your metabolism that occurs when you cut calories too low is equivalent to about one-third of the amount of calories you have cut. In other words, if the average 63.5 kg (10 stone) woman, goes on a 1,000-calorie a day diet (which means cutting 1,000 calories a day from her recommended daily amount of 2,000), her metabolism will slow by roughly 333 calories, meaning only 667 of those calories actually contribute to her weight loss. Cutting calories too low doesn't work.

It teaches you to eat properly

When most of us come to the end of a standard diet, the first thing we do is go out and eat all those foods we've been missing, which often starts the needle on the scales moving upwards again. On this diet you've been eating those favourite foods all along, so there's no making up to be done. More importantly, by following the weekend eating guidelines you learn how to control yourself around these foods – and how to enjoy them without feeling guilty – forever.

What to expect

What we eat and the amount of exercise we do affects our bodies in many, many different ways – from our appearance to the way we feel and the overall health of our bodies. Changing your diet – even if it is only from Monday to Friday – and your usual exercise will therefore cause changes in your body.

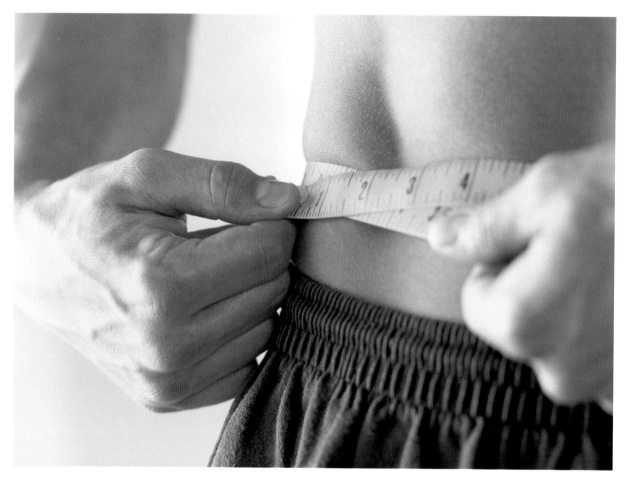

Weight loss

The average weight loss on this diet is 0.5–1 kg (1–2 lb) a week. In a world where other diets claim you can lose 3 kg (7 lb) over seven days this might not sound much, but losing weight slowly and steadily maximizes the chance that what you are losing is actually fat and not just water or muscle. This isn't just healthier for your body, it also makes it more likely that you'll keep the weight off as the more muscle you have in your body, the higher your metabolism.

Inch loss

This won't just happen because you're losing weight. You'll probably be doing more exercise on this plan than normal and it's this that will tone up your muscles and help boost the inches you lose as the weight comes off. If you're already a regular exerciser you might be tempted to skip the workouts in this book, but don't. The muscles in the body respond to change – if you do the same workout over and over again it stops challenging your body and you stop getting results. Think about adding some of the toning moves (see pages 80–99) to your daily schedule and you'll give your body an extra shake-up.

Improved energy levels

One of the main elements of this diet is the fact that you eat little and often so as to speed up your metabolism, but this isn't the only positive effect that eating in this way has on your body. Grazing on regular, small, balanced meals also helps prevent sudden falls in your blood sugar, which lead to the fatigue and mood swings that plague most of us and which can trigger diet-busting cravings mid-afternoon as we aim to increase our energy through sugary foods. The effects are so fast that by day three or four on this plan you should notice that your afternoon energy dips and sugar cravings have disappeared – and that they go for good.

Increased vitamin intake

Research from Scotland's Queen Margaret's University, Edinburgh, found that people who eat little and often have higher levels of nutrients in their diets than those who eat three square meals a day. This was particularly true of vitamin C, which the body can't store in large amounts and which is a major immunity-boosting vitamin. Getting enough of this vitamin in your diet can result in much less severe versions of colds and flu if you do get them.

Improved general health

Your general health will receive a boost not only from the extra vitamins you're taking in, but also from your increased activity as a result of following the exercise plans in this book. It is now widely recognized that regular exercise can help reduce the risk of cancer and heart disease, strengthen bones, boost mood and dramatically cut the risk of depression.

Improved hair, skin and nails

When most of us go on a slimming diet these are the areas that suffer as we take away essential fats that help keep skin hydrated, reduce our calcium intake by cutting down on dairy foods which makes nails suffer, and often forgo the healthy proteins hair needs in order to grow. Levels of all of these are actually increased on this plan.

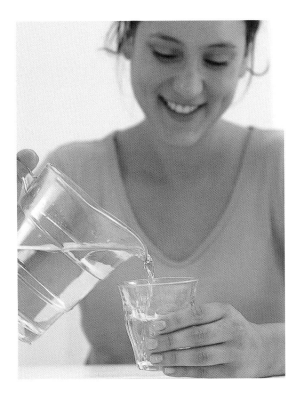

A possible side effect

The diet menus in this book are high in fibre-filled foods like fruit and vegetables. For most people this will bring only positive effects since fibre is a major health booster, preventing problems like constipation and fatigue and generally improving the health of the digestive system. For others, however, suddenly increasing fibre intake can lead to extra gas in the digestive system and associated bloating and discomfort. If this happens to you, don't quit the plan. Instead, cook vegetables for a little longer and chew them well to help digestion. Also, make sure you're drinking about eight glasses of water every day to help keep food moving through your body. If you know that certain vegetables trigger a bloating reaction, it's fine to swap them for other vegetables that suit your digestive system better. Finally, if you do get gassy, drinking peppermint tea can help calm things.

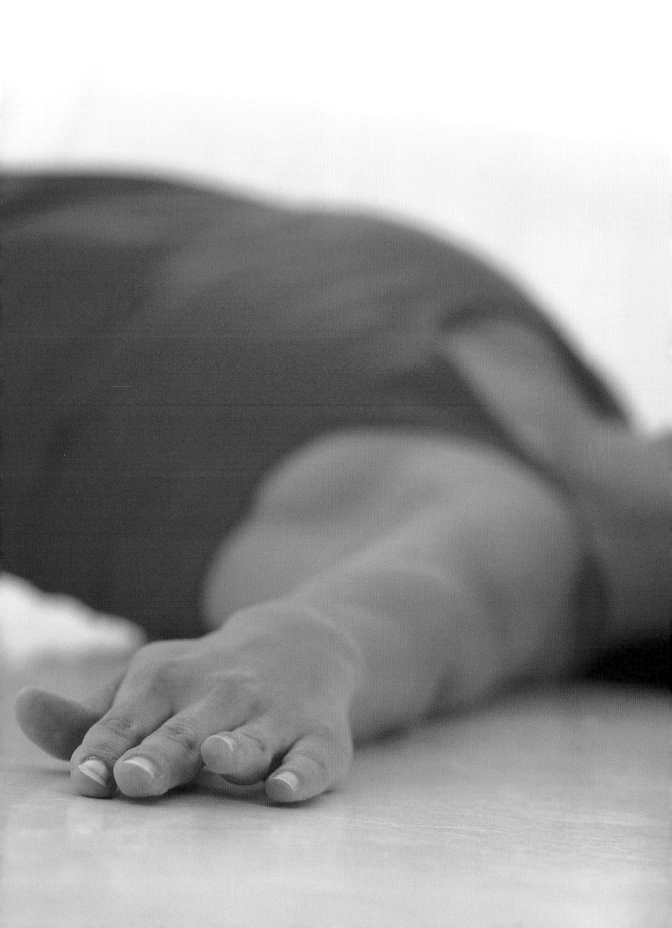

your
metabolism

Diets work by creating a difference between the number of calories you take in each day and the number you burn up. While most diet plans focus only on the former by cutting calorie intake, this diet also maximizes the latter by boosting the speed at which your body naturally burns calories. This is known as your metabolic rate, or metabolism.

On the following pages you'll discover how hard your metabolic rate is likely to be working (which will help you tailor the diet plans in this book to your personal needs), you'll find out which foods speed up metabolism, and how these and certain exercises can ensure you start burning calories even when you're sitting still.

What is metabolism?

Metabolic rate is the amount of energy, measured in calories (or kiloJoules), that the body uses up each day. The total figure for this comes from three different sources: the calories we burn when moving about, those we burn when digesting food and, finally, those the body burns everyday simply keeping all our systems working – known as the resting metabolic rate.

Resting metabolic rate

Every single task that the body carries out each day to keep us alive and thriving – such as breathing, thinking, fighting off germs and bugs, and repairing cells – burns lots of energy. Unless you're a very heavy exerciser, your resting metabolic rate accounts for the majority – 60–70 per cent – of your total calories burnt every single day. However, just as height, weight and hair colour differ from person to person, so, too, does this resting metabolic rate. How fast or slow is your metabolism is determined by a number of different factors. These can include genetics, gender and age.

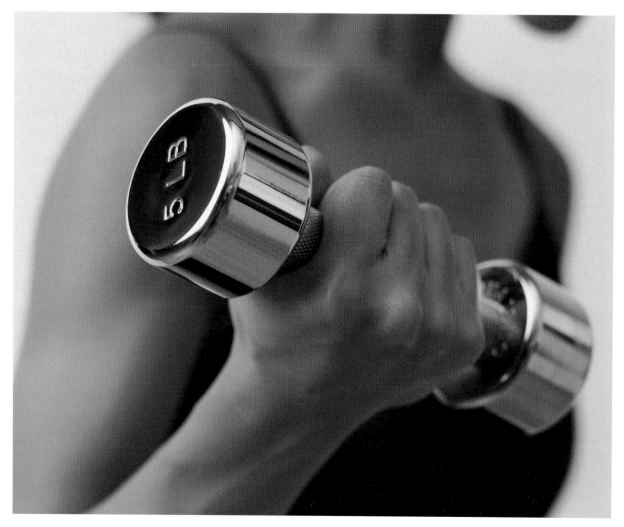

Genetics

It's estimated that 60 per cent of the speed of your metabolic rate is determined by your genes, as these control how much muscle you have in your body and how effectively your thyroid gland, which drives the metabolic rate, works. Studies on identical twins have shown that they have identical metabolic rates so, if your parents have a slow metabolic rate, so will you.

Gender

Men generally have slightly faster metabolisms than women, because they have lower levels of body fat and higher levels of muscle mass as part of their genetic make-up. This is important as muscle is what fitness experts refer to as 'metabolically active', which means that it actually burns calories to survive. This means that the more muscle you have in your body, the higher your metabolic rate.

Age

While male metabolism does slow with age, the decline is greater for women. From the age of about 35, the hormonal changes that occur in the female body to prepare it for menopause also start to affect the body's ability to retain muscle. As a result, each year in the 10–15 years before menopause the average woman loses roughly 0.25 kg (½ lb) of muscle. After menopause, when the hormone levels are lower, that loss doubles. This means that every decade women also see a fall in the amount of calories they burn each day. Prior to menopause, this fall is around 100 calories a day less than the figure burnt in a woman's twenties. Post-menopause, she could be burning 200–300 calories less per day. This slowdown is one of the primary reasons why weight gain often occurs in middle age.

Fitness

The above three factors may cause some of you to decide that in dietary terms you're doomed. However, there is a fourth factor that determines your resting metabolic rate – your fitness level. The more exercise you do, the more muscle you tend to have in your body – and the higher your metabolic rate. Every 0.5 kg (1 lb) of muscle you gain through exercise increases the number of calories you burn each day by about 50.

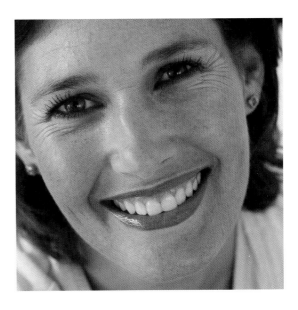

Could your thyroid be making you fat?

The thyroid is a tiny butterfly-shaped gland in your neck. If we regard muscle mass as the engine that powers metabolic rate, then the hormones released by the thyroid gland are the fuel that determines how fast it can drive. In most people the thyroid functions normally, but in about 3 per cent of us the thyroid stops producing adequate levels of hormones and the metabolism slows down, which is a condition called hypothyroidism. One side effect of this slowdown is weight gain, so if you really do find it impossible to lose weight on a very low-calorie diet and you suffer from more than two of the symptoms below to a significant degree (above about a six on a scale of one to ten), you may want to see your doctor for a thyroid check:

- Fatigue or lethargy
- Mood swings and irritability
- Feeling cold all the time
- Very dry skin or hair
- Thinning hair or eyebrows
- Aching joints
- Menstruation problems
- Constipation

Eating to boost metabolism

Digesting food is an energy-intensive process – chewing, producing digestive acids, moving things around the system and absorbing nutrients all takes effort. The result is that 5–10 per cent of our daily calorie expenditure is taken up simply by converting the food we eat into something we can use. We can use this process to boost weight loss.

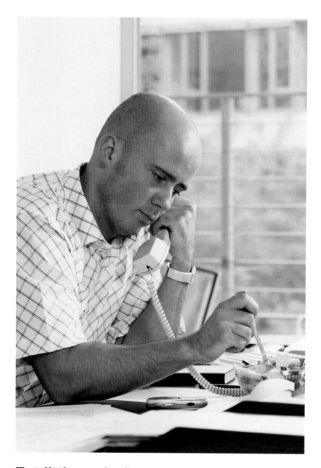

Eat little and often

Eating little and often is the key to losing weight successfully. This may go against what many of you have done in the past, but it really does help your metabolism and prevent the hunger pangs and sugar cravings that derail many normal diets.

The thermogenic boost

Trials at the University of Massachusetts in the US have found that people who eat more than four times a day have a 45 per cent less chance of being overweight than those who eat less than three times a day. The reason for this is that all those tasks involved in digesting even the smallest intake of food mean that every single time you eat, you burn calories doing it, and this 'thermogenic' boost (as it's known to scientists) lasts for 2–3 hours after the food has left your mouth. If you therefore switch from the traditional eating pattern of three square meals a day to one where you're eating three moderate meals a day plus two or three snacks your body is constantly in 'digestion' mode, and constantly running at a higher metabolic rate. This helps increase that vital calorie difference between what you take in each day and what you use up, and improves your weight loss results. But this isn't the only way it helps.

Metabolically active muscle is retained

Japanese researchers at Nagoya University put two sets of dieters on the same diet of 1,200 calories a day, but asked one set to eat them in two large meals and the other set to have six mini meals (known as grazing) throughout the day. Their results showed that the grazers were found to have lost more body fat and retained more muscle than those eating the larger meals. This is explained by the fact that a dieting body burns both stored muscle and stored fat for energy but, if you drop calories too low and leave too long between meals, the 'starving' body goes into self-preservation mode and protects its fat stores, therefore using up a greater proportion of muscle than fat as fuel for energy. Remember, muscle is metabolically active so it is desirable to retain muscle mass. The more muscle you have in your body the more calories you burn each and every day, and the more weight you lose because of it.

Balanced sugar levels

Grazing also works because it stops you craving diet-busting foods like chocolate, confectionery and sugar. Our body produces energy from the food we eat by turning it into the sugar glucose that it finds easy to use as fuel. When levels of glucose are balanced in the blood the body is happy, but if these sugar levels plummet it starts to panic and sends out signals that we need more glucose – and fast. To you, these panic signals feel like sugar cravings and the next thing you know, you're eating chocolate and your diet is doomed.

There are two main reasons why glucose levels can fall – you leave too long between meals, or you eat too large a meal in one go, which causes a surge of glucose in the blood that the body then also panics over, shuttling it rapidly into the fat/muscle stores. Eating little and often, however, prevents both these potential sugar disrupters and keeps your energy on an even keel.

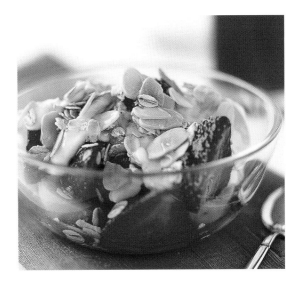

Breakfast: the most important metabolic meal of the day

You'll notice that breakfast on this diet is a big deal – there's cereal, toast, eggs, there's even pancakes if you want them. This is because when it comes to metabolic boosting, breakfast is the most important meal you can eat. Overnight our metabolic rate slows down by about 5 per cent, and without the thermogenic kickstart provided by breakfast your body can be running at this slower rate until lunch. It might not sound much but that measly 5 per cent slowdown could account for a weight gain of 1.2 kg (2½ lb) every single year! The fact is that regular breakfast eaters have above-average metabolic rates, while breakfast skippers have lower-than-average ones. This is one of the most fundamental reasons why, on average, early eaters weigh 3.6 kg (8 lb) less than those who skip their morning meal.

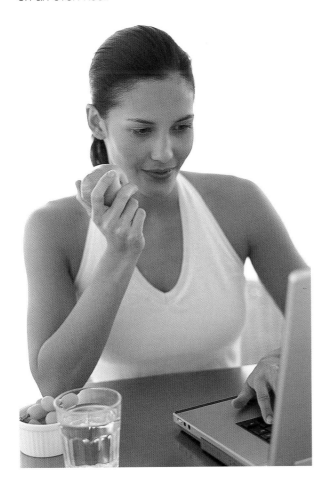

Foods that boost metabolism

While all foods trigger thermogenesis, certain foods can accentuate its effects by causing chemical changes in the body that raise metabolism further or trigger the body's fat-release mechanism. These foods provide the basis of the diet you'll be following from Monday to Friday each week. Expect to eat at least three servings of metabolism-boosting foods a day.

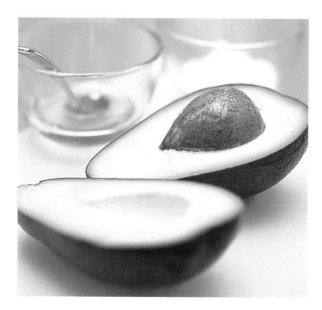

Avocados

The essential fats found in avocados actually rev up metabolic rate, speeding fat burning. Avocados are also the primary food source of a vital liver-boosting antioxidant called glutathione, and it's the liver that controls how fast fat is burnt in your body.

Breakfast cereals

Our bodies have to work hard to break down fibre. Every gram of fibre eaten takes 7 calories (29 kJ) to process, so eating more high-fibre foods like breakfast cereals (particularly those with bran or oats) aids weight loss.

Chilli pepper

Chilli (and potentially other hot spices like cayenne, curry and ginger) causes the release of the hormone adrenalin, which increases metabolic rate by roughly 25 per cent. Chilli is also an appetite suppressant, helping you feel fuller after each meal.

Dairy products

Researchers at the University of Tennessee in the US found that calcium, particularly that occurring in dairy products, has the ability to switch fat cells from storage mode to burning mode, thereby increasing weight loss. In addition, it inhibits the production of new fat cells, cutting the risk of weight regain.

Dried fruit

Dried fruit is high in iron, which is essential in metabolic terms. When iron levels are low your whole body slows down, including the rate at which you burn calories. Iron is also responsible for retaining adequate blood oxygen levels and, just as fire can't burn without oxygen, neither can fat.

Grapefruit

Grapefruit lowers levels of the fat storage hormone insulin, helping promote fat burning. The effects are so great that recent US research from San Diego's Scripps Clinic found that having half a grapefruit or a glass of grapefruit juice before meals caused volunteers to lose 4.5 kg (10 lb) in three months, without changing any other part of their diet.

Green tea

According to Swiss researchers at the University of Geneva, drinking five cups of green tea a day increases metabolism by about five per cent, which could potentially trigger a weight loss of 3.6 kg (8 lb) a year.

Lean proteins (fish, chicken, turkey, lean red meat)

Of all the food types, your body finds it hardest to digest proteins. After eating a high-protein meal or

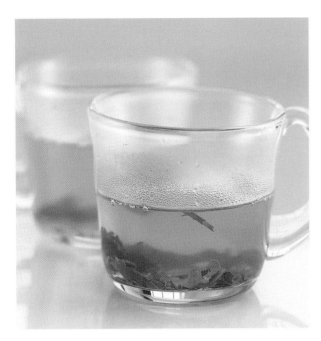

snack your metabolism therefore runs 20–30 per cent faster than normal. Protein also has the highest satiety of the food groups, meaning that you feel fuller sooner.

In addition, red meat is an important source of iron and of a healthy fat called conjugated linoleic acid, which helps preserve muscle and release body fat.

Nuts

Nuts are high in protein and essential fats, and just one handful can increase metabolism by around 11 per cent. Nuts are also important for satiety, so eating them as snacks can reduce the amount you eat at your next meal.

Olives and olive oils

These are also important sources of metabolism-boosting essential fats so don't be afraid to eat them in moderation. Studies from Harvard Medical School in the US reveal that people who do so are at least 5 kg (11 lb) thinner than those who shun fat completely.

Pears

While only three per cent of people have a medically defined slow thyroid (see page 17), many other people may have a slightly sluggish one (affected by age, diet and female hormones). Iodine helps boost thyroid function – and pears are one of the richest and most easily accessible sources of the mineral.

Soya foods

Research at the University of Utah in the US found that animals fed on soya-based feeds had half the body fat of those fed other diets; epidemiological research indicates a similar trend in people. It's believed that the isoflavones (which mimic the female hormone oestrogen) in soya help suppress fat storage.

Water and water-filled foods

According to recent German trials in Berlin's Humboldt University, within 40 minutes of drinking a glass of water, the rate at which the average person burns calories increases by 30 per cent – and stays this way for more than an hour. In fact, every glass of water you drink actually burns 25 calories because of this metabolic boost.

Similarly, University of Utah researchers found that dehydration causes metabolic rate to slow down by two to three per cent. Around 40 per cent of the fluid we take in each day comes from food – but you can increase this further with water-filled foods like melon, cucumber, celery and lettuce.

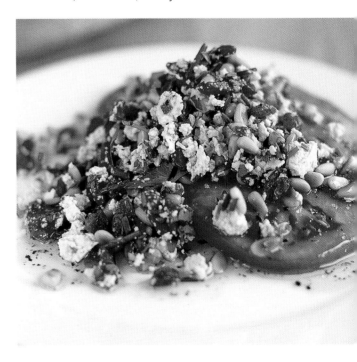

Exercise and metabolism

Exercise is a major metabolism booster. At its simplest level, it works because movement burns calories. For the average person, 20–30 per cent of the energy used up each day is burnt via movements like walking to the bathroom or fridge, by more intense exercise like jogging, gym workouts or team sports, and even by movements you're unaware of such as fidgeting.

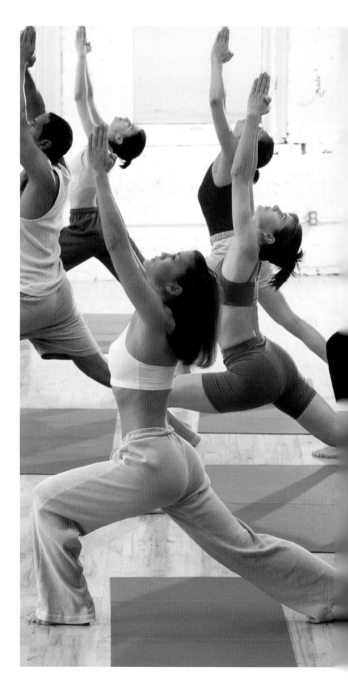

Age is no barrier

It doesn't matter how old you are, exercise can still boost your metabolism. In trials at the University of Alabama in the US, 15 people in their sixties and seventies were put on a strength training programme three days a week. At the end of the six-month trial, they were burning 230 calories a day more due to increased muscle mass and the extra burst of energy their bodies had post-workout.

The body furnace

Since muscle is metabolically active and burns calories simply by existing, the more muscle you have, the more calories you burn. All exercise increases muscle mass to some degree, but the best type of workouts for building muscle are strength training workouts where you lift external weights or your own body weight. Lifting weights puts pressure on your muscles and helps them grow. In the long term this boosts metabolism by increasing the amount of muscle you have, but it also has an important short-term effect.

The way in which exercise makes us stronger is by creating tiny little tears in the muscle, which the body then repairs – just as it does a cut in your skin. This rebuilding, combined with the extra oxygen, blood and other fluids flowing in and out of the muscles post-exercise, all keep your body revved up well after your workout is over. According

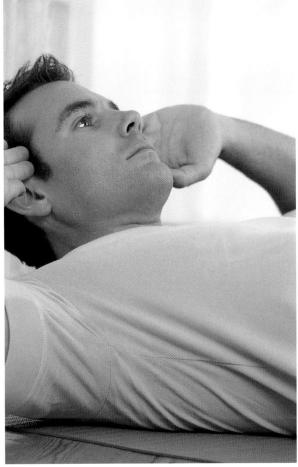

to research in the journal *Medicine & Science in Sports & Exercise*, after a good workout you can be burning calories up to 30 per cent faster for up to 2 hours afterwards, and this can play a further part in maximizing your weight loss.

Keep exercising

Ultimately, if you want to lose weight and keep it off, you should be exercising and there's plenty of advice in this book to help you do it. If the idea scares you, immediately makes you feel time pressured, or just sends you into 'but I hate exercise mode', it shouldn't. The strength training plans in this book (see pages 80–83) take only 8–10 minutes a day to complete (plus a quick warm-up and cool-down). And the aerobic exercises – the ones when you burn the most calories actually doing the workouts (see page 96–99) – can be fitted into the busiest day and offer possibilities for even the most strident exercise hater.

Three metabolism myths busted

Myth 1
Fatter people have slower metabolisms
While metabolism does vary from person to person, not every fat person has a slow metabolism. In fact, the more you weigh, the more calories you actually burn up moving around and carrying out essential tasks like breathing so your metabolic rate is actually higher than that of a thin person.

Myth 2
Yo-yo dieting slows your metabolic rate
While your metabolism does slow down after a few days on a diet (one of the reasons for the cyclic approach of this diet), when you come off the diet and stop restricting calories it fires back up again. However, if you've been crash dieting and losing more than 1 kg (2 lb) a week (especially if you weren't exercising) you will have lost muscle while you slimmed, which will reduce the calories you burn each day.

Myth 3
Pregnancy slows down metabolism.
Although most women do gain weight while pregnant and find it hard to lose afterwards, nothing happens hormonally during pregnancy that slows metabolic rate. After giving birth, however, mothers who breastfeed experience a raised metabolic rate, resulting in an increased calorie burn of around 500 calories a day.

Assess your metabolic rate

Knowing whether you have an above- or below-average metabolic rate may be useful if you are trying to lose weight. The quiz below helps you estimate how fast or slow your metabolism is likely to be running right now – and gives you some pointers on how this might affect your weight-loss efforts.

What to do

Look at the statements below and tick all those to which you would answer 'yes'.

☐ I am male

☐ I am aged under 30*

☐ I am aged under 50*

☐ I lift weights more than three times a week*

☐ I lift weights five or more times a week*

☐ People often tell me to stop fidgeting

☐ I never skip meals

☐ my job has some active element like walking or lifting

☐ I drink more than 2 litres (3½ pints) of water a day

☐ I rarely feel cold

☐ I always eat breakfast

☐ my leg muscles are fairly well defined

☐ I run/cycle/swim or do fast aerobic work of some kind most days

☐ my abdominal muscles are fairly well defined

☐ I walk for at least 30 minutes a day (not necessarily all in one go)

☐ I stand up as part of my job for at least 2 hours a day

☐ I very rarely watch television in the evenings

☐ I have never crash dieted

☐ when I have lost weight in the past I have kept it off

☐ I do eat the wrong things quite often and deserve to have gained more weight than I actually have

☐ I sleep more than 6 hours a night

☐ I do toning and firming exercises at an exercise class or at home to a video

☐ I have not gone through the menopause

* With these statements, tick them both if both apply to you. For example, if you are 27 years old you are both under 30 *and* under 50, so tick both statements. Similarly, if you lift weights six days a week this means you also weightlift more than three days a week, so again tick both statements.

Results

Count up the number of ticks you've marked above then read the relevant paragraph below to determine what it might mean.

9 or less

You probably have a slower-than-average metabolism. The chances are that you find it very easy to put on weight and hard to take – or keep – it off. While some of this may be down to age and/or gender, most problems occur because of your diet and exercise habits, which are slowing everything down. Building muscle mass will really help you, so give the toning plans (see pages 80–99) your maximum effort every day. If you have at least a basic level of fitness, you could even think about doing two toning workouts a day, although it's best to choose different routines to prevent overworking the same muscles. In addition, use simple metabolic boosts like green tea and extra chilli peppers to fire things up.

10–18

You probably have an average metabolism. You know that if you stick to a diet the weight will come off slowly – but it's the boredom of the slow weight loss that stops you succeeding with your aims. Because of this, weekends could be the danger time for you on this diet: while someone with a fast metabolism may be able to burn off any extra calories that sneak into their diet, with an average metabolism there's more risk of indulgences adding up. This doesn't mean you don't take weekends off dieting, just that you should really follow the rules closely (see pages 104–113) and watch out for problems like mindless eating or oversized portions that can cause excess calories to creep in. Keeping a food diary at weekends will really help with this (see page 114).

19 or over

You probably have a high metabolism. Weight loss is actually fairly easy for you – but because you burn so many calories a day, diets can leave you hungry. Because the weekday plan on this diet is a balanced diet, this shouldn't happen here, but if you do start to get fatigued then you might actually need to add some more food each day.

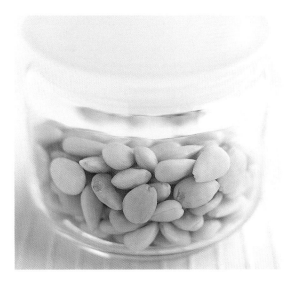

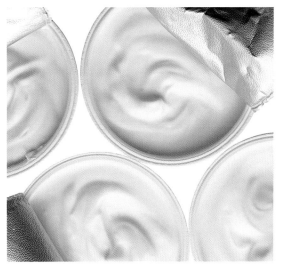

Safe snacking

Start with one more high-nutrient snack a day of around 100 calories, and if your problems continue – and you're still losing at least 0.5 kg (1 lb) a week – then try adding another one. Good snacks to choose would be any two pieces of fruit, one piece of fruit and five almonds or 50 g (2 oz) low-fat cottage cheese, 125 g (4 oz) pot soya or low-fat dairy yogurt, a handful of crudités with 3 tablespoons salsa, 75 g (3 oz) chicken or a hard-boiled egg or 150 ml (¼ pint) glass of skimmed milk with half a banana.

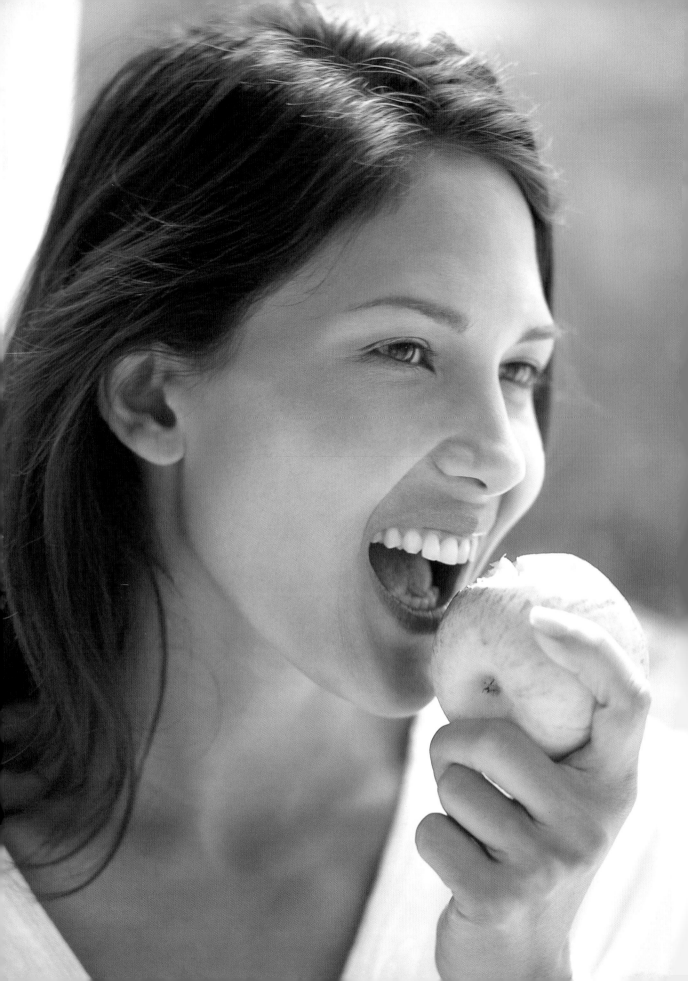

the weekday diet

Since your weekday eating habits are very structured on this diet, the following pages list exactly what you should eat from Monday to Friday each week. There are two plans available: one for non-vegetarians (see pages 30–51) and one for vegetarians (see pages 52–73). Each includes low-calorie, tasty recipes and easy alternatives for those who don't like to spend too long cooking. And don't worry about not having all the ingredients to hand – exactly what you need each day is clearly laid out for you.

Knowing what to eat on a diet plan is only part of losing weight. To truly succeed you need willpower to stick with it – and that's not always readily available. That's why motivation tips and reward ideas are a big part of this chapter – you can use these whenever you need them.

The weekday rules

Although the diet is incredibly flexible, there are still some rules that you have to stick to in order to make it work. Below are the five rules to follow from Monday to Friday. (See pages 104–113 for the weekend rules – don't worry, they're just as easy.)

The rules: Monday to Friday

1 Your weekend off is only Saturday and Sunday. It does not begin when you leave work Friday night and end with brunch on Monday morning!

2 Don't skip meals or snacks. Instead of increasing your weight loss, this will actually slow it down as you need to keep eating regularly.

3 Try to stick to the diet as directed. It's been carefully planned to provide the optimum level of calories for weight loss and nutrients for health. In addition, it incorporates high levels of metabolism-boosting foods (see pages 20–21) to maximize results.

4 If you do slip up at any point, don't fall into the 'all or nothing' trap. Get straight back on the plan with the next meal or snack – remember you have plenty of chances to eat treat foods at the weekend.

5 Don't skip the exercise section that starts on page 74. Working out can double or even triple the amount of weight you lose each week. Also, toning your muscles creates a firmer, slimmer, healthier body than can be achieved by weight loss alone.

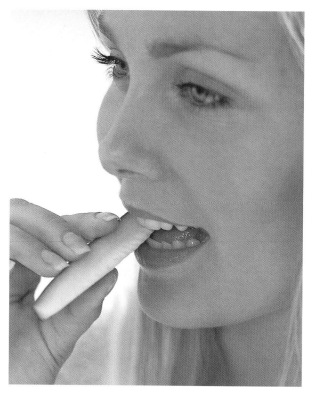

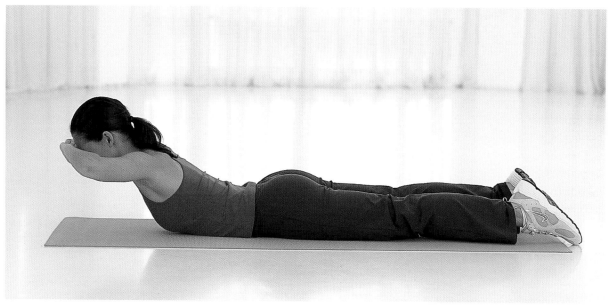

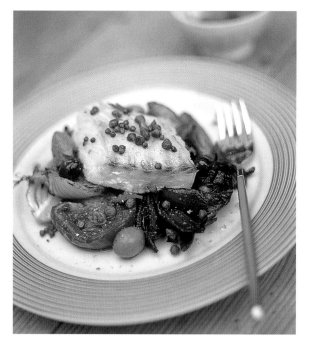

At the end of the fortnight...

Since the diet spans only two weeks, there are a number of options at the end of the fortnight. You can repeat the diet as is or repeat just some days; you can mix and match days from both plans (if you're a non-vegetarian) or start customizing the diet yourself by sticking to the same meals, but replacing like for like. For example, swap a fruit for another fruit; chicken for fish or lean pork; eggs for tofu, Quorn or soya mince; rice for pasta and so on.

Alternatively, start making up your own meals using a calorie chart. Aim for a breakfast of around 350 calories, a lunch of around 450 calories, dinner of around 500 calories and two snacks of 100 calories each. Do, however, try and stick to the rule of at least three metabolism-boosting foods a day in your menus.

Frequently asked questions

Q: I don't like some of the foods in the plan – what do I do?

You can swap like for like: for example, any fruit or vegetable on the plan can be swapped for an equivalent-sized serving of another fruit or vegetable (except potatoes). You can swap fish for chicken, turkey, lean red meat or shellfish, and vice versa. Carbohydrates are also interchangeable; if the recipe says rice and you don't like it, have pasta, couscous or noodles instead. Just don't leave out any food group.

Q: I eat out a lot for work – how does this fit into this plan?

The problem with restaurant eating is that you never really know what's gone into a dish, so calorie counting can be incredibly erratic. Also, portions are often larger than you'd serve yourself. However, order plain steak, chicken or fish served with a salad or vegetables; pasta served with any non-creamy sauce; salads with low-calorie dressing; or stir-fried dishes with plain rice, and you should be all right – particularly if you stop eating as soon as you feel full.

Q: What can I drink?

It's estimated that the average person consumes 14 per cent of their daily calories in the form of beverages. While you're following this diet, you should aim for 2 litres (3½ pints) no-calorie fluid a day. Water or green tea (see Quick tip, page 32) are best, but you can also have ordinary tea, plain coffee, herbal tea and diet soda. You can also have an allowance of up to 150 ml (¼ pint) skimmed milk a day for use in tea and coffee.

Q: I can't store food at work; can I still follow the diet?

Yes, the variety of meals suggested is to keep you interested, but if it's hard for you to pull out a chicken satay, for example, on your tea break, go for seven dried apricots, a small handful of any nuts or 125 g (4 oz) pot soya or low-fat dairy yogurt for each snack. At lunch, choose either six pieces of sushi or any less-than-300 calories ready-made sandwich, both accompanied by ready-made vegetable crudités (no dip except salsa) or any two pieces of fruit. Try to include at least one metabolism-boosting food (see pages 20–21) in the meal.

The weekday diet for non-vegetarians

Now you know the weekday rules, it's time to get started; but before you do, here's an explanation of the features you'll see on the diet plan each day. Don't ignore them. What you want to eat may seem more interesting, but each of these tips is to help you stay motivated or to make the diet easier for you in some way.

Motivation tips

While you probably won't go hungry on this plan, and the sheer variety and intense tastes of many of the recipes should stop you getting bored, the fact that you are sticking to an organized eating plan can still mean that there are days when you want to quit, or when cravings strike. The easiest way to deal with this is just to tell yourself that come Saturday you can eat anything you like, so you really don't need it now. If, however, you are still struggling, the motivation tips for each day should help keep you focused.

Daily rewards

Another way to boost motivation is to give yourself a treat each day. This gives your brain positive feedback, which not only helps you make healthy choices the next day, but also helps you break the habit of soothing negative feelings like stress, boredom or loneliness with food.

To use the reward tips, pick the one that's recommended that day or – particularly if you're a man who doesn't fancy painting his nails, for example – find one that appeals to you more on another page. Another good way to choose your reward is to spend a few minutes assessing your mood at the end of the day, then look through all the reward suggestions in the book and find one that aims to tackle those emotions best.

Daily shopping lists

There's nothing more frustrating than trying to follow a recipe and realizing halfway through that you're missing one of the main ingredients. This frustration doubles on a diet where all your meals are planned for you. That's why on each page you'll find a list of foods you need 'fresh' each day. This doesn't mean that you have to shop every day – 'fresh' is in quotation marks for a reason. A lot of the foods in the plan repeat from day to day so you can buy, for example, seven tomatoes and a huge bag of baby spinach at the beginning of the week and not have to buy any more that week. Each night after dinner, or first thing in the morning, quickly check the ingredients you need for the day ahead. If you're running low, stock up accordingly.

There are some foods not on this 'fresh' list. These are the so-called storecupboard (or basic fridge-stored) foods, which you probably already have, or that you can buy on day one of the diet and keep until required. The box opposite lists the items you'll need on the non-vegetarian diet plan.

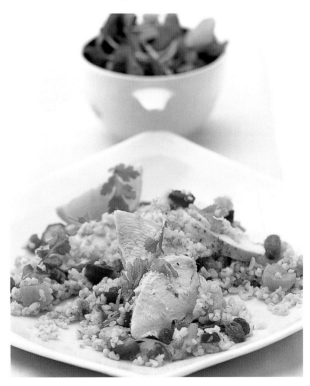

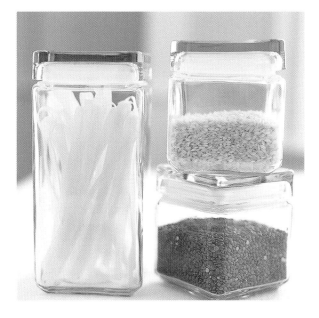

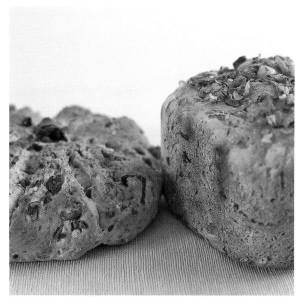

Storecupboard essentials for non-vegetarians

Main ingredients
- Bran or other high-fibre breakfast cereal
- Porridge oats
- Almonds (in their skins – see Quick tip, page 66)
- Walnuts
- Pumpkin seeds
- Sunflower seeds
- Dried apricots
- Canned fish: tuna in brine or spring water, salmon and/or sardines in tomato sauce
- Canned tomatoes
- Canned slimmer's vegetable soup and/or miso soup sachets (see Quick tip, page 36)
- Canned lentil soup
- Canned grapefruit segments in natural juice (unless using fresh)
- Green tea (see Quick tip, page 32)
- Granary or wholemeal bread
- Basmati rice
- Lentils (dried or canned)
- Couscous
- Self-raising flour (white and wholemeal)
- Oatcakes or crispbreads
- Dried pasta (such as penne or fusilli)

Herbs, spices and condiments
- Peanut butter
- Salsa
- Low-calorie mayonnaise
- Low-calorie dressing
- Mustard (any type except honey mustard)
- Extra-virgin olive oil
- Balsamic vinegar
- Soy sauce
- Curry powder
- Hot chilli pepper sauce
- Sweet chilli sauce
- Honey
- Head of garlic
- Fresh lemon juice
- Salt and freshly ground black pepper

In the fridge
- Eggs
- Skimmed milk
- Low-fat yogurt or fromage frais (natural or fruit-flavoured)
- Low-fat cream cheese
- Low-fat cooking spread
- Grapefruit juice

Today's plan

⭐ Reward yourself ⭐

Apply a face pack. Not only will this make your skin look healthier, it's also a good way to tackle any urges to nibble in front of the television. You can't eat with a face pack on – especially if you choose a clay mask that hardens as it works, and they make these for men, too!

Choose blue...

The meals on this diet plan are designed so you shouldn't be hungry, but if your plate looks empty you can feel psychologically hungry. This is when your brain decides it needs more food even though your stomach is full! Beat this by switching to a smaller plate – especially if you choose a blue one since blue is an inhibiting colour that suppresses appetite.

If you really do feel hungry, then it's okay to add very low-calorie foods like lettuce, bean sprouts, alfalfa, spinach, celery or cucumber to any meal.

Quick tip

To liven up green tea, or disguise the taste if you find it too bitter, add 1 teaspoon freshly squeezed lemon juice or honey, or a splash of orange juice.

Breakfast

50 g (2 oz) **bran cereal** served with 150 ml (¼ pint) skimmed milk, or **porridge** made from 50 g (2 oz) porridge oats mixed as per the instructions with a little water, plus 150 ml (¼ pint) skimmed milk to drink. Top your choice of cereal with 1 chopped **banana** and 2 handfuls of fresh or frozen **strawberries** (or other berries such as blueberries, blackberries, raspberries, or red or blackcurrants).

Also make yourself a cup of metabolism-boosting **green tea** – aim for five cups today and every day on the plan.

Mid-morning snack

1 **pear** and 10 **almonds** plus 125 g (4 oz) pot **low-fat yogurt**.

Lunch

Option ❶ **Tuna niçoise-style salad** made from unlimited green beans, tomatoes and red onions, topped with 75 g (3 oz) tuna (canned in brine or spring water), 10 pitted olives and 1 hard-boiled egg; 150 ml (¼ pint) glass of **grapefruit juice.**

Option ❷ Sandwich made with 2 slices of **granary or wholemeal bread**, 75 g (3 oz) **tuna** (canned in brine or spring water) or **cooked chicken**, and **low-calorie mayonnaise** or **mustard**, served with a **side salad** of your choice, dressed with a **low-calorie dressing** or a squeeze of fresh **lemon juice**.

Afternoon snack

1 small **pitta bread** or 1 slice of **granary or wholemeal toast** served with 2 tablespoons **salsa** and a small plate of **vegetable crudités** (such as sticks of carrot, cucumber and celery).

Dinner

125 g (4 oz) lean **sirloin steak** served with **Watermelon and Feta Salad** (see page 33) and 150 g (5 oz) **new potatoes**.

Watermelon and Feta Salad

preparation time 10 minutes **cooking time** 2 minutes **serves** 4
Kcal 99 (416 kJ) **Protein** 3 g **Carbohydrate** 9 g **Fat** 6 g

1 tablespoon black sesame seeds
500 g (1 lb) watermelon, peeled, deseeded and diced
175 g (6 oz) feta cheese, diced
2½ handfuls of rocket
handful of mint
2 tablespoons olive oil
juice of ½ large lemon
salt and freshly ground black pepper

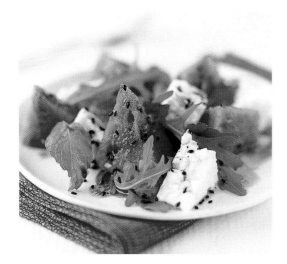

watermelon and Feta Salad

❶ Dry-fry the sesame seeds for a few minutes until aromatic, then set aside. Arrange the watermelon and feta cheese on a large serving plate with the rocket and mint.

❷ Whisk together the olive oil and lemon juice, then season to taste with salt and pepper. Drizzle over the salad, scatter over the sesame seeds and serve.

Buy fresh today

- Banana
- Berries (fresh or frozen)
- Pear
- Green beans, tomatoes, red onions and olives (for lunch option 1)
- Carrots
- Cucumber
- Celery
- Watermelon
- Rocket
- New potatoes
- Mint
- Sirloin steak
- Cooked chicken plus salad vegetables (for lunch option 2)
- Feta cheese (preferably reduced-fat)
- Pitta bread, white or wholemeal (if using)
- Black sesame seeds

Today's plan

Breakfast

Smoothie made from 1 **banana**, 2 handfuls of fresh or frozen **blueberries** (or other berries such as blackberries, strawberries, raspberries, or red or blackcurrants) and 150 ml (¼ pint) **skimmed milk**; 2 slices of **granary or wholemeal toast**, each topped with 1 teaspoon **peanut butter** or 2 teaspoons **low-fat cream cheese**.

Mid-morning snack

3 **celery** sticks topped with 25 g (1 oz) **feta cheese** or **low-fat soft cheese**.

Lunch

200 g (7 oz) **baked potato** topped with 75 g (3 oz) **tuna** (canned in brine or spring water) mixed with ¼ **red chilli**, finely chopped, (optional) and 2 teaspoons **low-calorie mayonnaise** or 3 tablespoons **salsa**. Serve with sliced **cucumber** and **green peppers**.

Afternoon snack

125 g (4 oz) pot **low-fat yogurt** or **fromage frais**.

Dinner

Option ❶ **Chicken Satay** (see page 35; ideally this should be marinated so prepare it in advance) served with 50 g (2 oz) dry weight **basmati rice** and 1 tablespoon **sweet chilli sauce** or **salsa**, plus unlimited **mangetouts** or **sugar snap peas.**

Option ❷ 4 sticks store-bought **chicken satay** or 150 g (5 oz) plain **chicken** breast, grilled and served with 50 g (2 oz) dry weight **basmati rice**, 1 tablespoon **sweet chilli sauce** and unlimited **mangetouts**; 1 piece of **fruit.**

Reward yourself

Treat yourself to an early night. Not only will you feel rested and refreshed, a good night's sleep also lowers levels of the stress hormone cortisol in your body. This is beneficial to dieting because cortisol causes fat storage.

Positive thinking...

Spend a minute today telling yourself you really can lose all the weight you want to on this diet. According to research published in the US's NUTRITION RESEARCH NEWSLETTER, this increases the success of a diet by 40 per cent. A good phrase to repeat to yourself is: 'Today I'm going to make the healthy choices that will help me to lose my weight.'

Quick tip

A 200 g (7 oz) potato is about the size of a tennis ball. If you're ordering your potato from a sandwich bar, ask for a small potato.

Chicken Satay

preparation time 10 minutes, plus marinating **cooking time** 10 minutes **makes** 10 sticks

Kcal 82 (344 kJ) **Protein** 13 g **Carbohydrate** 1.5 g **Fat** 3 g

25 g (1 oz) smooth peanut butter

125 ml (4 fl oz) soy sauce

125 ml (4 fl oz) lime juice

15 g (½ oz) curry powder

2 garlic cloves, chopped

1 teaspoon hot chilli pepper sauce

500 g (1 lb) chicken breast, cut into roughly 50 cubes

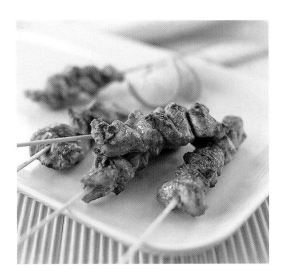

Chicken Satay

1 In a large mixing bowl combine the peanut butter, soy sauce, lime juice, curry powder, garlic and hot chilli pepper sauce.

2 Place the cubes of chicken in the marinade, cover well and leave to marinate for about 12 hours (or overnight) in the fridge.

3 When ready to cook, spear the chicken on to 10 skewers, with roughly 5 cubes per stick. Cook for 5 minutes on each side under a preheated high grill. Serve hot, setting aside 2 skewers in the refrigerator as a snack for tomorrow.

Buy fresh today

- Banana
- Berries (fresh or frozen)
- Celery
- Potato
- Cucumber
- Green pepper
- mangetouts or sugar snap peas
- Fruit of your choice
- Red chilli (if using)
- Chicken breasts or ready-made chicken satay
- Feta cheese (preferably reduced-fat) or low-fat soft cheese
- Bottled lime juice (or about 5 fresh limes)

Today's plan

Breakfast
Porridge made from 50 g (2 oz) porridge oats mixed as per the instructions with a little water. Add 1 chopped **apple** and 4 chopped **dried apricots**. 150 ml (¼ pint) glass of **skimmed milk.**

Mid-morning snack
2 **chicken satay** sticks (leftover from yesterday) or 3 slices of **smoked chicken** (available from the deli counter), plus ½ **grapefruit** or 6 **canned grapefruit segments**.

Lunch
6 pieces of store-bought **seaweed-wrapped sushi**, plus a bowl of **miso soup** or 200 g (7 oz) can any brand of slimmer's **vegetable soup.**

Afternoon snack
1 **pear**, chopped and dipped in 1 teaspoon **peanut butter** or 50 g (2 oz) **low-fat cottage cheese.**

Dinner
Option **1** **Puy Lentils with Flaked Salmon and Dill** (see page 37), served with a **rocket salad** dressed with **balsamic vinegar.**
Option **2** 125 g (4 oz) **salmon steak,** grilled and served with 200 g (7 oz) **canned lentils** and 50 g (2 oz) frozen/fresh weight **peas.**

Quick tips
- Unlike many beans and pulses, dried lentils don't require soaking before use and they cook quickly, readily disintegrating to a mush. Puy lentils are a small, good-quality French variety.

- Miso is a paste fermented from soya beans, which is widely used in oriental cooking for flavouring soups, marinades and sauces. Miso soup, which contains the miso paste along with tofu, wakame seaweed and various vegetables, is available by the sachet in supermarkets and oriental stores.

Reward yourself
Phone someone you've not spoken to for a while – spend at least 10 minutes pacing backwards and forwards while you talk and you'll burn off an extra 50 calories at least.

Keep a willpower diary...
Every time you beat a food craving, you go for a walk when you don't really want to or you turn down a sweet treat, write it down. When you're struggling with your diet, read this to yourself to remind yourself of the strength of your willpower.

Puy Lentils with Flaked Salmon and Dill

preparation time 30 minutes **cooking time** 30–40 minutes **serves** 4
Kcal 447 (1877 kJ) **Protein** 42 g **Carbohydrate** 18 g **Fat** 21 g

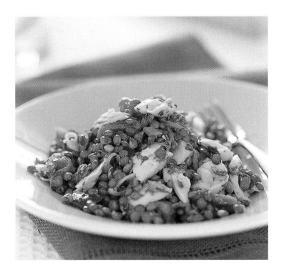

Puy Lentils with Flaked Salmon and Dill

500 g (1 lb) salmon tail fillet
2 tablespoons dry white wine
4 red peppers, halved, cored and deseeded
175 g (6 oz) Puy lentils, well rinsed
large handful of dill, chopped
1 bunch of spring onions, finely sliced
lemon juice, for squeezing
freshly ground black pepper

Dressing
2 garlic cloves, peeled
large handful of flat-leaf parsley
large handful of dill, roughly chopped
1 teaspoon Dijon mustard
2 green chillies, deseeded and roughly chopped
juice of 2 large lemons
1 tablespoon olive oil

1 Place the salmon on a sheet of foil and spoon over the wine. Gather up the foil and fold over at the top to seal. Place on a baking sheet and bake in a preheated oven, 200°C (400°F), Gas Mark 6, for 15–20 minutes. Allow to cool before flaking.

2 Meanwhile, flatten the pepper halves slightly. Grill, skin side up, under a preheated hot grill for a few minutes until charred. Enclose in a plastic bag for a few minutes to allow them to soften, then peel away the skin and cut the flesh into 2.5 cm (1 in) cubes, reserving any juices.

3 Place all the dressing ingredients except the oil, in a food processor or blender and process until smooth. Still processing, drizzle in the oil until the mixture is thick.

4 Place the lentils in a large saucepan with plenty of water, bring to the boil, then simmer gently for 15–20 minutes. Drain and place in a bowl with the red pepper, dill, spring onions and black pepper to taste.

5 Stir the dressing into the hot lentils and allow to infuse. Add the flaked salmon and mix through. Squeeze over the lemon juice and serve.

Buy fresh today

- Apple
- Grapefruit (fresh or canned)
- Pear
- Red peppers, spring onions, green chillies, fresh dill and flat-leaf parsley and rocket (for dinner option 1)
- Peas (fresh or frozen) (for dinner option 2)
- Smoked chicken (if using)
- Salmon
- Low-fat cottage cheese
- Sushi
- Dry white wine (for dinner option 1)

Today's plan

Reward yourself

Give yourself a hand massage (or, better still, get someone else to do it!). It's a great way to relieve stress.

1 Cover your hands with some massage oil or hand cream.

2 Squeezing fairly tightly, rub from your wrist down to your fingers about five times, then gently rub between each finger and thumb.

3 Now massage each of your fingers in turn with quick strokes from base to tip. Repeat the first squeezing movement then swap hands.

Shop carefully...

When doing your supermarket shop, try to avoid the centre aisles. These tend to be the ones with sugary or fatty treats in them – most healthy food tends to be around the outside.

Breakfast
½ grapefruit or 6 **canned grapefruit segments**; 2 **eggs**, poached or scrambled, 2 halved and grilled **tomatoes** and 1 slice of **granary or wholemeal toast.**

Mid-morning snack
1 large slice (around one-eighth of a whole fruit) of **watermelon** and 25 g (1 oz) **feta cheese.**

Lunch
3 slices of **cooked chicken** served with a salad of **rocket** and **red pepper**, topped with ¼ **avocado**, 6 **almonds** and 4 **dried apricots**, all chopped. Drizzle with **lemon juice** and 2 teaspoons **olive oil.**

Afternoon snack
125 g (4 oz) pot **low-fat yogurt** plus 2 handfuls of fresh or frozen **raspberries** (or other berries such as blueberries, blackberries, strawberries, or red or blackcurrants) and 1 **banana.**

Dinner
Option **1** **Couscous with Grilled Vegetables** (see page 39).
Option **2** 125 g (4 oz) **chicken breast** or **fish fillet**, grilled and served with 50 g (2 oz) dry weight **couscous** and unlimited **broccoli.**

Quick tip
Salads like this lunchtime version can be prepared the night before and stored in the fridge. Just add the lemon juice and oil at the last minute to prevent the ingredients going soggy.

Couscous with Grilled Vegetables

preparation time 10 minutes **cooking time** 10 minutes **serves** 4
Kcal 470 (1974 kJ) **Protein** 12 g **Carbohydrate** 85 g **Fat** 8 g

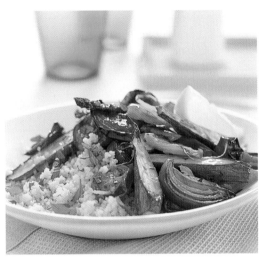

Couscous with Grilled Vegetables

300 g (10 oz) couscous
500 ml (17 fl oz) boiling water
2 red peppers, cored, deseeded and quartered
1 orange pepper, cored, deseeded and quartered
6 baby courgettes, halved lengthways
2 red onions, cut into wedges
24 cherry tomatoes
2 garlic cloves, finely sliced
2 tablespoons olive oil
125 g (4 oz) asparagus spears
grated rind and juice of 1 lemon
4 tablespoons chopped herbs (such as parsley or mint)
salt and freshly ground black pepper

1 Tip the couscous into a large bowl, pour over the water, cover and set aside while preparing the remaining ingredients.

2 Place the peppers, courgettes, onions, tomatoes and garlic in a grill pan in a single layer. Drizzle with the oil and cook under a preheated hot grill for 5–6 minutes, turning the vegetables occasionally.

3 Add the asparagus to the grill pan and continue to grill for 2–3 minutes until the vegetables are tender and lightly charred. When the peppers are cool enough to handle, remove the skins and discard.

4 Fork through the couscous to separate the grains. Toss with the grilled vegetables, lemon rind and juice and herbs. Season to taste with salt and pepper and serve.

Buy fresh today

- Grapefruit (fresh or canned)
- Tomatoes
- Watermelon
- Feta cheese (preferably reduced-fat)
- Cooked chicken
- Rocket
- Red pepper
- Avocado
- Berries (fresh or frozen)
- Banana
- Orange pepper, baby courgettes, red onions, cherry tomatoes, asparagus, lemon and fresh herbs (for dinner option 1)
- Chicken breast or fish (for dinner option 2)
- Broccoli (for dinner option 2)

Today's plan

Breakfast

Option ❶ **Pear Pancakes** (see page 41).
Option ❷ 2 **crumpets** or 2 slices of **granary or wholemeal bread**, toasted, each topped with 1 teaspoon **peanut butter** or 2 teaspoons **low-fat cream cheese**, plus 1 sliced **pear**; 150 ml (¼ pint) **skimmed milk**, to drink.

Mid-morning snack

4 **dried apricots** and 25 g (1 oz) **feta cheese** or 50 g (2 oz) **low-fat cottage cheese**.

Lunch

Sandwich made with 2 slices of **granary or wholemeal bread**, 1 **hard-boiled egg**, mashed and mixed with 1 teaspoon **low-calorie mayonnaise**, 1 sliced **tomato** and a few **rocket** leaves. Serve with 10 black, green or mixed **olives** and a few **celery** sticks.

Afternoon snack

1 **banana** and 150 ml (¼ pint) **skimmed milk**, blended into a smoothie if you like, plus 6 **almonds**.

Dinner

125 g (4 oz) lean **pork chop** served with 150 g (5 oz) uncooked weight **sweet potato**, boiled and mashed or baked, plus unlimited **broccoli**.

Reward yourself

Buy yourself something new this weekend – it needn't be expensive. A book, a DVD, or something cosmetic like nail polish or aftershave will work. If you can, try to choose something with orange in the packaging. It's the colour of motivation and energy so it might also help you focus.

Quick tip

If you are always short of time in the morning, you can speed things up by making the pancake mixture the night before, storing it in the fridge and starting the recipe at Step 2 instead. It's also quicker if you make 1 large pancake per person, rather than 3 small ones.

Give yourself an emotion audit...

Friday nights can trigger comfort eating as we either reward ourselves for a good week or commiserate over a bad one. Stop cravings by asking yourself what is really the matter and specifically treating that emotion. For example, if you're stressed have a relaxing bath.

Pear Pancakes

preparation time 10 minutes **cooking time** 20 minutes **serves** 4 (makes 12 small pancakes or 4 large ones)
Kcal 378 (1585 kJ) **Protein** 10 g **Carbohydrate** 52 g **Fat** 16 g

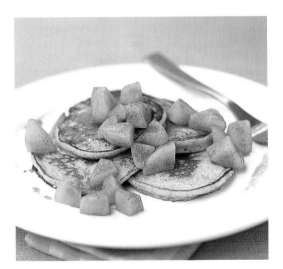

Pear Pancakes

50 g (2 oz) low-fat cooking spread, melted
50 g (2 oz) self-raising flour
50 g (2 oz) wholemeal self-raising flour
25 g (1 oz) porridge oats
1 tablespoon caster sugar
2 eggs, lightly beaten
275 ml (9 fl oz) buttermilk
milk, for thinning (optional)
oil, for brushing
Pears
6 pears, peeled, cored and chopped
pinch of cinnamon
1 tablespoon water

1 In a bowl, beat the low-fat cooking spread, flours, oats, sugar, eggs and buttermilk together until smooth. Add a little milk if the mixture looks very thick.

2 Brush a nonstick frying pan with a little oil and heat. Add a ladleful of batter to the pan (or 3 ladlefuls if making larger pancakes) and cook for 2 minutes on each side until golden. Remove the pancake from the pan and keep warm while you make more pancakes using the remaining batter mixture.

3 Meanwhile, place the pears and cinnamon in a small saucepan with the water. Cover and cook gently for 2–3 minutes until just tender. Serve the pancakes, rolled or folded, accompanied by the cooked pears.

Buy fresh today

- Pears
- Tomato
- Rocket
- Celery
- Banana
- Sweet potato
- Broccoli
- Pork chop
- Feta cheese (preferably reduced-fat) or low-fat cottage cheese
- Buttermilk, caster sugar and cinnamon (for breakfast option 1) or crumpets (for breakfast option 2)
- Olives

Today's plan

Breakfast

Omelette made from 1 whole **egg** and 2 **egg whites** and filled with 1 chopped **tomato** and 50 g (2 oz) **reduced-fat cheddar**; 150 ml (¼ pint) glass of **grapefruit juice**.

Mid-morning snack

2 **crispbreads** or **oatcakes** topped with ¼ **avocado**, mashed, or 2 teaspoons **low-fat cream cheese**.

Reward yourself

Take a long relaxing bath tonight. If you can fill it with a bubble bath or oil containing orange or grapefruit, this is even better, since both of these help stimulate fat burning.

Wake up and think positive...

The success of the weekend-off idea depends on you getting straight back on your diet first thing Monday morning. Switch on your motivation by thinking of five diet successes you had last week – or, if things were tough, by making a list of five things that losing the weight will help you do – and focus on these.

Lunch

Option ❶ Pasta and pesto salad: Cook 50 g (2 oz) dried penne and mix in 1 tablespoon pesto. Leave to cool (or refrigerate overnight) and, ideally, just before serving add 6 halved cherry tomatoes and 2 slices of lean ham, finely chopped. If you need to take this dish to work, you can add the ingredients in the morning, but keep the tomatoes whole. Serve with a side salad of **rocket** dressed with a little **balsamic vinegar.**
Option ❷ Sandwich made with 2 slices of **granary or wholemeal bread**, 2 slices of **lean ham, turkey** or **chicken** and **salad**; 25 g (1 oz) bag **reduced-fat potato crisps.**

Afternoon snack

125 g (4 oz) pot **low-fat yogurt** plus any piece of **fruit**.

Dinner

Option ❶ Tamarind and Lemon Grass Beef (see opposite) served with 50 g (2 oz) dry weight **basmati rice** and unlimited **broccoli.**
Option ❷ 150 g (5 oz) lean **sirloin steak,** grilled, served with 50 g (2 oz) dry weight **basmati rice** and a serving of **broccoli** or **green beans**. You can also spice things up with a splash of **salsa** or **hot chilli pepper sauce** on top of the rice.

Quick tip

Tamarind paste is a sticky brown paste commonly used in Indonesian and Thai cooking to provide a slightly tart or sour taste. You'll find it in most large supermarkets and Asian stores, or you can order it online from many specialist cook's stores.

Tamarind and Lemon Grass Beef

preparation time 15 minutes **cooking time** 12 minutes **serves** 4
Kcal 265 (1113 kJ) **Protein** 28 g **Carbohydrate** 13.5 g **Fat** 10 g

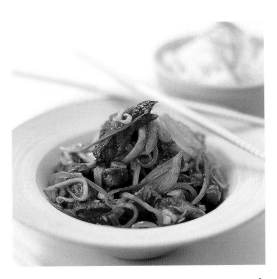

Tamarind and Lemon Grass Beef

1 tablespoon olive oil
500 g (1 lb) lean beef, cut into strips
2 stalks lemon grass, chopped
6 shallots, chopped
2 green chillies, chopped
3 tablespoons tamarind paste
2 tablespoons lime juice
2 teaspoons fish sauce
2 teaspoons brown sugar
200 g (7 oz) shredded green papaya

❶ Heat the oil over a high heat in a wok or frying pan. Toss in the meat and cook for 2–3 minutes.

❷ Add the lemon grass, shallots and chillies and stir-fry for a further 5 minutes or until the meat is well browned.

❸ Add the tamarind paste, lime juice, fish sauce, sugar and green papaya and stir-fry for a further 4 minutes before serving with rice.

Buy fresh today

- Tomato
- Avocado (if using)
- Cherry tomatoes and rocket (for lunch option 1)
- Fruit of your choice
- Broccoli or green beans
- Shallots, green papaya, lemon grass and green chillies (for dinner option 1)
- Lean beef (for dinner option 1) or sirloin steak (for dinner option 2)
- Lean ham (for lunch option 1) or lean ham, turkey or chicken (for lunch option 2)
- Reduced-fat cheddar
- Reduced-fat potato crisps (for lunch option 2)
- Pesto, preferably reduced-fat (for lunch option 1)
- Tamarind paste, bottled lime juice (or 1 lime), fish sauce and brown sugar (for dinner option 1)

Today's plan

Reward yourself

Sit down with a good book or your favourite magazine. Not only is this a treat, it can help distract you from a food craving, most of which last only 10 minutes, and you'll be able to tick off another success in your willpower diary. Do avoid reading while you're eating though – it takes your focus off how your body is feeling and you may find you eat too much.

Quick tips

● It might seem strange to eat fruit and chicken together but the combination really does work and the added protein from the chicken helps you feel fuller than you would after a snack of fruit alone.

● If you don't like the slightly bitter taste of walnuts, you can replace them with an equivalent amount of almonds, or try 1 tablespoon porridge oats instead.

Breakfast

Option ❶ **Walnut and Banana Sunrise Smoothie** (see page 45) with 1 slice of **granary or wholemeal toast** topped with 1 teaspoon **peanut butter** or 2 teaspoons **low-fat cream cheese**.

Option ❷ 1 handful of **almonds** or other nuts, 2 slices of **granary or wholemeal toast** topped with 1 mashed **banana**; 150 ml (¼ pint) **skimmed milk**.

Mid-morning snack

1 large slice (around one-eighth of a whole fruit) of **watermelon** or 2 pieces of any other **fruit**; 3 slices of **smoked chicken or turkey** (available from the deli counter).

Lunch

Small **pitta bread** or 1 slice of **granary or wholemeal bread** served as an 'open sandwich', filled with 15 g (½ oz) **low-fat cream cheese**, 50 g (2 oz) **lean ham** and sliced **tomato**. Serve with 3 tablespoons **salsa** and unlimited **vegetable crudités** (such as sticks of carrot, cucumber and celery).

Afternoon snack

6 **almonds**.

Dinner

150 g (5 oz) **salmon** or **tuna** fillet served with 50 g (2 oz) **dried fusilli** (pasta spirals) topped with 3 tablespoons **Spicy Tomato Sauce** (see page 45).

Find some role models...

Go online and find some weight-loss chat rooms. Reading about their successes can really help you stick at things.

Walnut and Banana Sunrise Smoothie

preparation time 5 minutes **serves** 2

Kcal 265 (1113 kJ) **Protein** 10 g **Carbohydrate** 35 g **Fat:** 11 g

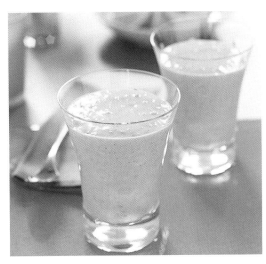

1 orange, segmented

1 banana

150 ml (¼ pint) skimmed milk

150 g (5 oz) natural yogurt

25 g (1 oz) walnut pieces

❶ Place all the ingredients in a food processor or blender and process until smooth and frothy. Pour into 2 glasses and serve.

walnut and Banana Sunrise Smoothie

Spicy Tomato Sauce

preparation time 5 minutes **cooking time** 15 minutes **serves** 4

Kcal: 49 (206 kJ) **Protein:** 1.5 g **Carbohydrate:** 2.5 g **Fat:** 0.1 g

400 g (13 oz) can chopped tomatoes

1 onion, chopped

1 garlic clove, crushed

2 tablespoons chopped basil

1 teaspoon dried rosemary

1 small red chilli (optional)

125 ml (4 fl oz) red wine (optional)

❶ Place all the ingredients in a saucepan and simmer, uncovered, for 15 minutes.

❷ Remove from the heat and allow to cool for 2–3 minutes, then transfer to a food processor or blender and process until smooth.

Buy fresh today

- Orange (for breakfast option 1)
- Banana
- watermelon or 2 fruits of your choice
- Tomato
- Carrot
- Cucumber
- Celery
- Onion
- Fresh basil
- Red chilli (if using)
- Smoked chicken or turkey
- Lean ham
- Salmon or tuna
- Low-fat cream cheese
- Pitta bread, white or wholemeal (if using)
- Dried rosemary
- Red wine

Today's plan

Breakfast

Any 3 pieces/slices of fruit (try **watermelon**, **pear** and **banana**) served with 125 g (4 oz) pot **low-fat yogurt** or **fromage frais**.

Mid-morning snack

Avocado roll-ups made from 2 slices of smoked turkey, ham or chicken spread with a little mustard, salsa or sweet chilli sauce and wrapped around ¼ avocado, cut into 2 slices.

Lunch

400 g (13 oz) serving of **tomato, vegetable or lentil soup** – store-bought or homemade – served with 2 slices of **granary or wholemeal bread** topped with 2 oz (50 g) **low-fat soft cheese**, 5 sliced **olives** and 1 sliced **tomato**.

Afternoon snack

6 **almonds** and 4 **dried apricots**.

Dinner

Option ❶ **Asparagus and Prosciutto Wraps** (see page 47) served with 150 g (5 oz) **new potatoes** and 2 **tomatoes**, halved and grilled.

Option ❷ 150 g (5 oz) **gammon steak** served with 150 g (5 oz) **new potatoes**, 2 halved and grilled **tomatoes** and 6 **asparagus spears**.

Reward yourself

Paint your nails. It's very hard to nibble food with wet nails – plus, if you paint them a bright colour it can even prevent overeating once the polish has dried. Most of us nibble unconsciously, but with a bright colour on your hands you're more aware of the movement of bringing your hand to your mouth – and this will make it easier to stop yourself.

Cook your vegetables al dente...

It's been shown that dieters find vegetables most satisfying if they are cooked al dente as they take longer to chew. This helps the brain send fullness signals to your stomach, making you feel fuller quicker.

Quick tip

Replace the prosciutto with Parma ham or rashers of streaky bacon if you prefer.

Asparagus and Prosciutto Wraps

preparation time 10 minutes **cooking time** 25–30 minutes **serves** 3

Kcal 415 (1743 kJ) **Protein** 43 g **Carbohydrate** 2.5 g **Fat:** 26 g

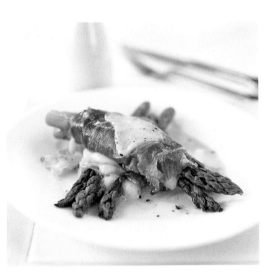

18 thick, fresh asparagus spears, trimmed

250 g (8 oz) prosciutto, thinly sliced

250 g (8 oz) mozzarella, cut into 18 equal slices

75 g (3 oz) butter, plus a little extra for greasing

freshly ground black pepper

Asparagus and Prosciutto Wraps

1 Plunge the asparagus spears into a large saucepan of boiling salted water and cook over a medium heat for 4–8 minutes or until the asparagus is tender but still crunchy. Drain and plunge into cool water. When the spears have cooled, drain once again and set aside.

2 Separate the prosciutto into 6 even piles. Take 3 asparagus spears and place them on 1 slice of prosciutto. Put 2 pieces of mozzarella in between the spears along with a small knob of butter. Wrap the prosciutto around the asparagus, using all the slices in the pile. Repeat until you have 6 bundles.

3 Arrange the asparagus bundles over the base of a lightly greased ovenproof dish. Place a slice of mozzarella and a knob of butter on each bundle. Season with black pepper and bake at the top of a preheated oven, 200°C (400°F), Gas Mark 6, for about 20 minutes.

Buy fresh today

- Fruits of your choice
- Avocado
- Tomatoes
- Asparagus
- New potatoes
- Smoked turkey, ham or chicken
- Prosciutto or alternative (for dinner option 1) or gammon steak (for dinner option 2)
- Low-fat soft cheese
- Mozzarella and butter (for dinner option 1)
- Olives

Today's plan

Reward yourself

Book a massage or sauna. Not only are these two great ways to fight the stress that can trigger comfort eating, both will help flush out any extra fluid that could add some extra weight on the scales tomorrow.

Keep dining rooms bright...

Research from the University of California in the US found that people eat more in dark rooms. The theory is that if you can't really see what you're eating your inhibitions become lower and you feel that what you are eating doesn't really count – but unfortunately it will when you come to weigh yourself tomorrow!

Quick tip

Open sandwiches are a great way to make you feel as if you're eating large amounts of food but for the same number of calories as a normal sandwich. If you eat them with a knife and fork (a good idea if you pile the toppings high) they feel even more like a meal.

Breakfast

Option ❶ High-Protein Muesli (see opposite) served with 150 ml (¼ pint) skimmed milk; ½ grapefruit or 6 canned grapefruit segments.

Option ❷ 50 g (2 oz) bran cereal served with 150 ml (¼ pint) skimmed milk and topped with 3 chopped dried apricots, 6 almonds and 1 chopped banana.

Mid-morning snack

2 pieces of any fruit.

Lunch

2 'open sandwiches' made with 2 slices of granary or wholemeal bread (ideally toasted) topped with 75 g (3 oz) canned salmon or sardines in tomato sauce, slices of cucumber and a few rocket leaves. Serve with sliced carrot, green pepper and celery.

Afternoon snack

15 olives and 1 oz (25 g) feta cheese or a low-fat cheese.

Dinner

125 g (4 oz) lean sirloin steak served with 150 g (5 oz) baked potato and a portion of Ratatouille (see page 49) or 200 g (7 oz) of a canned version.

High-Protein Muesli

preparation time 5 minutes **serves** 6
Kcal 500 (2100 kJ) **Protein** 14.5 g **Carbohydrate** 55 g **Fat** 24 g

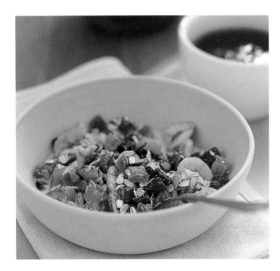

High-Protein Muesli

250 g (8 oz) porridge/rolled oats

100 g (3½ oz) pumpkin seeds

100 g (3½ oz) sunflower seeds

200 g (7 oz) ready-to-eat mixed dried fruit (such as apricots, figs, raisins, blueberries, pineapple, banana, peaches and papaya), chopped

6 brazil nuts, chopped

6 walnuts, chopped

1 Mix all the ingredients together and store in an airtight container in a cool dark place.

Buy fresh today

- Grapefruit, fresh or canned (for breakfast option 1) or banana (for breakfast option 2)
- Fruits of your choice
- Cucumber
- Rocket
- Carrot
- Green pepper
- Celery
- Potato
- Aubergines, Spanish onion, beef tomatoes and fresh basil (or canned ratatouille)
- Sirloin steak
- Feta cheese (preferably reduced-fat) or a low-fat cheese
- Olives
- Mixed dried fruit and brazil nuts (for breakfast option 1)

Ratatouille

preparation time 15 minutes **cooking time** 25–30 minutes **serves** 4
Kcal: 44 (186 kJ) **Protein:** 1.4 g **Carbohydrate:** 4.8 g **Fat:** 0.6 g

½ tablespoon olive oil

375 g (12 oz) aubergines, cut into 1 cm (½ in) chunks

½ large Spanish onion, cut into 1 cm (½ in) chunks

2 celery sticks, coarsely chopped

2 large beef tomatoes, skinned and deseeded

½ teaspoon chopped basil

1 Heat the oil in a nonstick frying pan until very hot. Add the aubergine and fry for about 10–15 minutes until very soft.

2 Place the onion and celery in a saucepan with a little water. Cook for 3–5 minutes until tender but still firm. Add the tomatoes and basil, then add the aubergine. Cook for 15 minutes, stirring occasionally.

Today's plan

Breakfast
Porridge made from 50 g (2 oz) porridge oats mixed as per the instructions with a little water. Add 1 chopped **banana** and 1 handful of fresh or frozen **blackberries** (or other berries such as blueberries, strawberries, raspberries, or red or blackcurrants).

Reward yourself
Have friends round for dinner. Tonight's recipe can easily be made to feed six or even eight people simply by increasing the amount of each ingredient you use. It's a great one to choose as it's so tasty that no one will think you're dieting – and it'll reinforce the idea that losing weight needn't be hard. If you want to offer your guests a dessert, a platter of fresh fruit would be ideal.

Mid-morning snack
½ **grapefruit** or 6 **canned grapefruit segments** and 6 **almonds**.

Lunch
1 **flour tortilla** (or 2 slices of **granary or wholemeal bread**) topped with ¼ **avocado**, mashed, 75 g (3 oz) **prawns** or **cooked chicken**, a sprinkling of chopped fresh red or green **chilli** (optional), and rolled into a wrap. Serve with a salad made from sliced **tomato**, **celery** and 15 **olives**.

Afternoon snack
125 g (4 oz) pot **low-fat yogurt**.

Dinner
Option ❶ **Pork with Chinese Cabbage** (see page 51), served with 50 g (2 oz) dry weight **basmati rice**.
Option ❷ A simple stir-fry of 75 g (3 oz) **lean pork**, **beef** or **chicken** with **red peppers**, **mangetouts** and **bean sprouts**. Serve with 1 tablespoon **sweet chilli sauce** on a bed of 50 g (2 oz) dry weight **basmati rice**.

Quick tip
To roll up a wrap, put the filling slightly to the right of centre of the tortilla, with about a 5 cm (2 in) gap all round the edge. Fold a large flap from the bottom over the filling. Now fold the right side of the tortilla and tuck it over and 'under' your filling. Now fold the left side over the right.

Get on the scales...
There's nothing more motivating than a good result on the scales, but don't weigh yourself every day. A once-weekly weigh-in, first thing in the morning after visiting the toilet, is the best plan. Friday morning, after four days on the diet, is a good day to check your weight and a good result will help you stay focused over the weekend ahead.

Pork with Chinese Cabbage

preparation time 5 minutes **cooking time** 40 minutes **serves** 4

Kcal 360 (1512 kJ) **Protein** 18 g **Carbohydrate** 8 g **Fat** 28 g

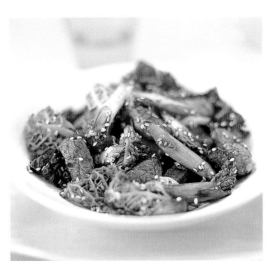

Pork with Chinese Cabbage

1 tablespoon white sesame seeds

2 garlic cloves, very finely sliced

3 spring onions, diagonally sliced into 1.5 cm (¾ in) pieces

½ teaspoon cayenne pepper

300 g (10 oz) pork loin, cut into thick strips

2 tablespoons olive oil

2 tablespoons sesame oil

2 tablespoons soy sauce

2 teaspoons honey

400 g (13 oz) Savoy cabbage, cut into strips

1 Toast the sesame seeds in a dry pan over a medium heat for 1–2 minutes or until golden brown, shaking continuously. Remove to a cool plate then set aside.

2 Combine the garlic, spring onions and cayenne pepper, then add to the pork, making sure the meat and flavourings are well combined.

3 Heat the oils in a frying pan and stir-fry the pork over a high heat, in about 3 batches, cooking for about 5 minutes on each side until golden and cooked through. Remove the meat from the pan and set aside. Add the soy sauce, honey and cabbage to the pan and toss to mix. Cover and cook over a medium heat for 5–6 minutes.

4 Return the pork to the pan, add the reserved sesame seeds, toss well and serve immediately.

Buy fresh today

- Banana
- Berries (fresh or frozen)
- Grapefruit (fresh or canned)
- Avocado
- Tomato
- Celery
- Spring onions and Savoy cabbage (for dinner option 1)
- Red peppers, mangetouts and bean sprouts (for dinner option 2)
- Red or green chilli (if using)
- Pork loin (for dinner option 1) or lean pork, beef or chicken (for dinner option 2)
- Prawns or cooked chicken
- Flour tortilla (if using)
- Olives
- White sesame seeds, cayenne pepper and sesame oil (for dinner option 1)

The weekday diet for vegetarians

The following pages give the weekday diet menus designed specifically for vegetarians. Don't think you're not getting the same metabolic boost as those who eat meat. High-fibre, high-protein combinations like beans, pulses, nuts and seeds rev things up, while your calcium stores are boosted via an intake of dairy products or a combination of leafy green vegetables and calcium-enriched foods.

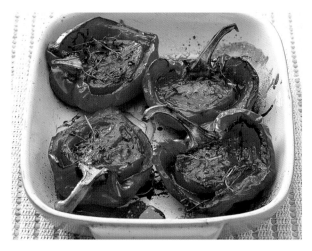

Motivation tips

It's one thing to know what foods to eat on a diet, but to lose weight you actually have to stick to them. As a vegetarian you have a natural advantage here – many of the foods that you obviously enjoy are already extremely diet friendly. However, this doesn't make it any easier to stick to an organized plan on days when comfort food is calling, or when sugary cravings strike.

That's why you'll find a motivation tip on every day of this plan to help you stay focused when times do get tough. Use these whenever you need them and always remember that, come the weekend, you can give in to any food cravings you might have so you really don't need to succumb now.

Daily rewards

Treats are also important motivation boosters, giving you non-food ways to soothe negative feelings like stress, boredom or loneliness. Every day you'll find a suggested way to treat yourself. How you use these is up to you. You can carry out one each night to keep you motivated or, every day, think about a particular challenge that you'll be facing (a birthday lunch, for example) and promise yourself that when you overcome that challenge you'll treat yourself to a reward – or even two! There are plenty of ideas on the non-vegetarian pages, too, so men should be able to find something suitable in case they don't fancy applying the fake tan or nail polish as suggested.

Daily shopping lists

One potential problem of being vegetarian (especially if you're a new convert) is that you may not make the most of the full variety of healthy foods available to you, causing you to rely too much on high-fat or high-sugar foods to stimulate your tastebuds. On this plan, however, you won't have these issues as the menus include a huge variety of foods, including an easy recipe to follow each day. This does take some organization, though, if you don't want to find suddenly, halfway through a recipe, that you don't have all the ingredients you need. That's why on each page you'll find a list of foods you need 'fresh' each day – and, some days, it might look quite long. However, don't panic – you don't have to try to fit in cooking, exercising *and* a trip to the shops each day. 'Fresh' is in those quotation marks for a reason. A lot of the foods in the plan repeat from day to day so you can buy, for example, onions and feta cheese at the beginning of the week and not have to buy any more that week.

There are some foods not on this 'fresh' list. These are the so-called storecupboard foods, which you probably already have, or that you can buy on day one of the diet and keep until required.

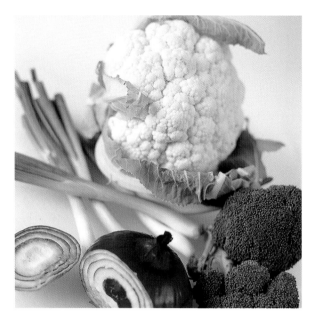
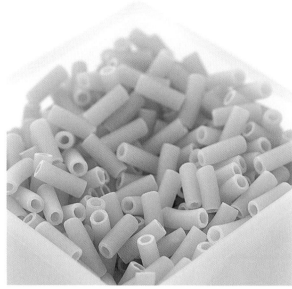

Storecupboard essentials for vegetarians

Main ingredients
- Bran or other high-fibre breakfast cereal
- Porridge oats
- Almonds (in their skins – see Quick tip, page 66)
- Walnuts
- Sunflower seeds
- Dried apricots
- Canned tomatoes
- Canned vegetable or lentil soup and/or miso soup sachets (see Quick tip, page 36)
- Green tea (see Quick tip, page 32)
- Granary or wholemeal bread
- Basmati rice
- Lentils (dried or canned)
- Couscous
- Self-raising flour (white and wholemeal)
- Oatcakes or crispbreads
- Dried pasta (such as penne or fusilli)
- Egg noodles

Herbs, spices and condiments
- Peanut butter
- Salsa
- Extra-virgin olive oil
- Balsamic vinegar
- Soy sauce
- Curry paste
- Hot chilli pepper sauce
- Sweet chilli sauce
- Honey
- Head of garlic
- Fresh lemon juice
- Vegetarian bouillon powder and/or stock cubes
- Salt and freshly ground black pepper

In the fridge
- Eggs
- Skimmed milk or calcium-enriched soya milk
- Soya or low-fat dairy yogurt or fromage frais (natural or fruit-flavoured)
- Low-fat cream cheese
- Butter, margarine or low-fat cooking spread
- Grapefruit juice

Today's plan

Reward yourself

Treat yourself to a foot soak. Green tea isn't just a great metabolic booster, it's also brilliant for soothing tired, achy feet (whether they're sore from stilettos or football boots). Pop 5 bags in a bowl of warm water and leave to steep for 5 minutes. Add some ice cubes then soak your feet for 5–10 minutes. Dry them well afterwards.

Quick tips

- Served as a dip or a spread, baba ganoush is made from smoked or chargrilled aubergines that have been puréed and combined with garlic, tahini (sesame seed paste), olive oil and lemon juice. You'll find it at the supermarket deli counter or in Middle Eastern food stores.

- Add hot chilli pepper sauces to dishes like pizza, pasta and soups for an extra metabolism boost.

Breakfast
50 g (2 oz) **bran cereal** served with 150 ml (¼ pint) **skimmed milk** or **calcium-enriched soya milk** and topped with 1 chopped **banana** and 2 handfuls of fresh or frozen **raspberries** (or other berries such as blueberries, blackberries, strawberries, or red or blackcurrants); **green tea** (see Quick tip, page 32) – aim for 5 cups today and every day on the plan.

Mid-morning snack
1 **pear** and 15 **almonds**.

Lunch
Sandwich made with 2 slices of **granary or wholemeal bread** and 50 g (2 oz) grated **reduced-fat cheese** or ½ **avocado**, sliced, plus 1 sliced **tomato**; 400 g (13 oz) serving of **lentil soup** – store-bought or homemade (see page 71).

Afternoon snack
3 tablespoons **baba ganoush** and a small plate of **carrot sticks**.

Dinner
Artichoke Pizza (see page 55) or 2 slices of any **thin crust vegetarian pizza** served with a large salad made from **baby spinach** and **cherry tomatoes,** dressed with **balsamic vinegar**.

Use the 'veggie' boost...

When researchers at Pennsylvania State University in the US asked people to eat two different meals, one high in vegetables, one low, the vegetable eaters felt fuller for longer. If ever you feel hungry, increase the portion sizes of vegetables in each dish.

Artichoke Pizza

preparation time 20 minutes **cooking time** 25–35 minutes **serves** 4
Kcal 293 (1233 kJ) **Protein** 4 g **Carbohydrate** 8 g **Fat** 10 g

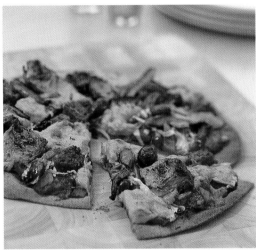

Artichoke Pizza

30 cm (12 in) ready-made pizza base

Tomato topping

400 g (13 oz) can tomatoes

1 onion, chopped

2 garlic cloves, chopped

1 teaspoon chopped oregano

1 green pepper, deseeded and chopped

1 red pepper, deseeded and chopped

1 carrot, grated

1 tablespoon olive oil

1 tablespoon balsamic vinegar

6 mushrooms, sliced

To garnish

6 canned artichoke hearts

black olives

6 strips of baked, smoked tofu

125 g (4 oz) reduced-fat cheddar or other hard cheese, grated (optional)

1 Place the canned tomatoes in a food processor or blender and process until smooth. Transfer to a large saucepan, add the onion, garlic and oregano and simmer gently for 20 minutes.

2 Stir the remaining tomato topping ingredients into the pan then pour the mixture over the pizza base, spreading it right to the edges. Arrange the garnish ingredients and cheese, if using, on top.

3 Place the pizza on a baking tray and cook in a preheated oven, 200°C (400°F), Gas Mark 6, for 5–10 minutes, or until the cheese starts to bubble and turn brown.

Buy fresh today

- Banana
- Berries (fresh or frozen)
- Pear
- Avocado or reduced-fat vegetarian cheese
- Tomato
- Carrots
- Onion, green and red pepper, mushrooms and fresh oregano (if making your own pizza)
- Baby spinach
- Cherry tomatoes
- Smoked tofu, reduced-fat vegetarian cheese, canned artichoke hearts and black olives (if making your own pizza)
- Baba ganoush
- Ready-made pizza base or ready-made thin-crust vegetarian pizza (depending on chosen option)

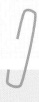

Today's plan

Reward yourself

Give yourself a fake tan. The real thing might not be healthy, but most of us feel more positive about our bodies when we have a tan – and feeling positive about the way you look helps increase diet results. The three tan rules to follow are:

1 Exfoliate and moisturize well before you start.

2 Wear gloves to stop you staining your palms.

3 Rub the fake tan in well as streaks occur when patches are left to dry unevenly on the skin.

Combat hunger with acupressure...

Acupressure can be useful for controlling stray hunger pangs. The appetite control point is on your ear, on the side closest to your head, just above the cartilage that runs across the middle of your ear. Here you'll find a little hollow. Use a cotton bud to gently press this point five to ten times whenever you feel hungry.

Breakfast
Walnut and Banana Sunrise Smoothie (see page 45 – replace the skimmed milk and yogurt in the recipe with soya-based alternatives if you don't use dairy products); 1 slice of **granary or wholemeal toast** topped with 1 teaspoon **honey** or **peanut butter**.

Mid-morning snack
1 large slice (around one-eighth of a whole fruit) of **watermelon** or 2 pieces of any other fruit, served with 50 g (2 oz) **low-fat cottage cheese** or 125 g (4 oz) pot **soya or low-fat dairy yogurt**.

Lunch
200 g (7 oz) **baked potato** (see Quick tip, page 34) topped with 2 tablespoons **baba ganoush**, served with a side salad made from **baby spinach**, grated **carrot** and **cherry tomatoes**.

Afternoon snack
2 **oatcakes** or **rye crispbreads** topped with ¼ **avocado**, mashed, or 2 teaspoons **low-fat cream cheese**.

Dinner
Vegetable Curry (see page 57) or any **reduced-fat vegetable curry ready meal** (under 300 calories) served with 50 g (2 oz) dry weight **basmati rice**.

Quick tip

Fruit is a healthy snack but because it's processed quickly through your digestive system it can leave you hungry soon after eating it. Adding cottage cheese or a soya yogurt to your snack helps keep you feeling fuller for longer.

Vegetable Curry

preparation time 10 minutes **cooking time** 20–25 minutes **serves** 4
Kcal 268 (1125 kJ) **Protein** 6 g **Carbohydrate** 35 g **Fat** 11 g

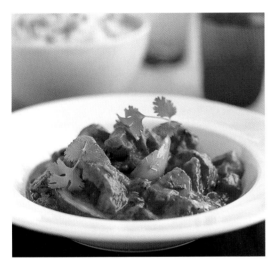

Vegetable Curry

1 tablespoon olive oil

1 onion, chopped

1 garlic clove, crushed

2 tablespoons medium curry paste

1.5 kg (3 lb) prepared mixed vegetables (such as courgette, pepper, mushrooms, green beans and potato – no more than 0.5 kg/1 lb of these)

200 g (7 oz) can chopped tomatoes

400 g (13 oz) can reduced-fat coconut milk

2 tablespoons chopped coriander leaves

1 Heat the oil in a large saucepan, add the onion and garlic and fry for 2 minutes. Stir in the curry paste and fry for 1 minute more.

2 Add the vegetables and fry for 2–3 minutes, stirring occasionally, then add the canned tomatoes and coconut milk. Stir well, bring to the boil, then lower the heat and simmer for 12–15 minutes until all the vegetables are cooked.

3 Stir in the coriander and serve.

Buy fresh today

- Orange
- Banana
- Watermelon
- Potatoes
- Baby spinach
- Carrot
- Cherry tomatoes
- Avocado (if using)
- Onion
- Vegetables such as courgettes, peppers, mushrooms and green beans (or a reduced-fat ready-made vegetable curry)
- Fresh coriander
- Low-fat cottage cheese
- Baba ganoush (see Quick tip, page 54)
- Reduced-fat canned coconut milk

Today's plan

Breakfast

2 slices of **granary or wholemeal toast,** each topped with ½ **banana**, mashed. Serve with a small handful of **almonds** and 150 ml (¼ pint) glass of **skimmed milk** or calcium-enriched soya milk.

Mid-morning snack

3 **celery** sticks topped with 25 g (1 oz) **feta cheese** or any **low-fat soft cheese** and dipped in 3 teaspoons **sweet chilli sauce**.

Lunch

6 pieces of store-bought **seaweed-wrapped vegetarian sushi rolls**, plus bowl of **miso soup** or 200 g (7 oz) can any brand of slimmer's **vegetarian soup**.

Afternoon snack

1 **apple** or **pear**, chopped into small pieces and mixed into 50 g (2 oz) **low-fat cottage cheese**. Serve with unlimited **carrot** sticks.

Dinner

Option ❶ **Hummus with Roasted Vegetables** (see page 59) served with 25 g (1 oz) dry weight **basmati or saffron rice.**
Option ❷ 1 **flour tortilla** topped with 2 tablespoons **reduced-fat hummus** or **baba ganoush**, spinach **leaves**, **red onion** and **tomato** and rolled into a wrap (see Quick tip, page 50). Serve with 50 g (2 oz) dry weight **basmati rice.**

Eat slowly and chew well...

It takes 20 minutes for your brain to register that your stomach is full, so eating slowly helps prevent overeating. In addition, the meals on this diet are very high in fibre so if you rush your food, your body may have trouble digesting it, which causes the bloating that makes you feel fat.

Reward yourself

Do something fun at lunchtime. Not only is having something to look forward to a good way to prevent boredom-related comfort eating, most of us rarely see sunlight in the middle of a 'work day'. However, researchers at Canada's University of British Columbia have found that sunlight helps cut carbohydrate cravings, so getting outside when you can could help you stay on track.

Quick tip

If you're not making your own hummus, watch the fat content carefully of store-bought versions. The healthiest brands of reduced-fat hummus have around 11–13 g or less fat per 100 g, most of it the healthy monounsaturated variety.

Hummus with Roasted Vegetables

preparation time 10 minutes **cooking time** 45 minutes **serves** 4

Kcal 422 (1783 kJ) **Protein** 16 g **Carbohydrate** 74 g **Fat** 9 g

8 small flour tortillas

Hummus

400 g (13 oz) can chickpeas, drained and rinsed

1 garlic clove

2 tablespoons Greek yogurt

juice of 1 lemon

pinch of paprika

Roasted vegetables

1 aubergine, cut into sticks

1 red pepper, cored, deseeded and sliced

2 courgettes, sliced

2 carrots, cut into sticks

1 red onion, sliced

1 tablespoon olive oil

1 teaspoon chopped thyme

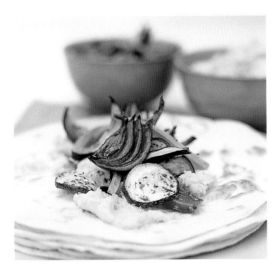

Hummus with Roasted Vegetables

1 To make the hummus, place the canned chickpeas, garlic, yogurt, lemon juice and paprika in a food processor or blender and process until smooth. Tip into a bowl, cover and set aside.

2 Place all the vegetables in a roasting tin, drizzle with the oil and sprinkle with the thyme. Cook in a preheated oven, 200°C (400°F), Gas Mark 6, for 45 minutes or until the vegetables are tender and just beginning to char.

3 Meanwhile, warm the tortillas according to the packet instructions, then fill with the roasted vegetables and hummus and serve.

Buy fresh today

- Banana
- Celery
- Apple or pear
- Carrots
- Aubergine, red pepper, courgettes and fresh thyme (for dinner option 1)
- Spinach leaves and tomato (for dinner option 2)
- Red onion
- Vegetarian feta cheese (preferably reduced-fat) or a low-fat soft cheese
- Low-fat cottage cheese
- Sushi
- Reduced-fat hummus or baba ganoush (see Quick tip, page 54)
- Flour tortillas
- Canned chickpeas, Greek yogurt and paprika (or ready-made reduced-fat hummus)

Today's plan

Breakfast

Option ❶ 50 g (2 oz) **bran cereal** and 6 chopped **dried apricots**, mixed into 125 g (4 oz) pot **soya or low-fat dairy yogurt**.

Option ❷ ½ **grapefruit** or 6 **canned grapefruit segments**; 2 **eggs**, poached or scrambled, and 2 halved and grilled **tomatoes**.

Mid-morning snack

1 **apple** and 6 **dried apricots**.

Lunch

1 small **pitta bread** spread with a little **salsa** and filled with 1 tablespoon **canned kidney beans**, 25 g (1 oz) **feta cheese** and ¼ **avocado**, chopped. Serve with 25 g (1 oz) bag **reduced-fat potato crisps**.

Afternoon snack

Smoothie made from 150 ml (¼ pint) **skimmed milk** or **calcium-enriched soya milk** and 3 handfuls of fresh or frozen **blueberries** (or other berries such as blackberries, strawberries, or raspberries, red or blackcurrants).

Dinner

Corn Fritters (see page 61) or a **Quorn steak** served with 75 g (3 oz) dry weight **red lentils** or 200 g (7 oz) **canned lentils**, unlimited **spinach** and a **tomato salad**.

Quick tip

If you don't eat eggs, soft tofu makes a great 'scramble'. Use about 125 g (4 oz) per person and cook it in a little butter or margarine as you would eggs. Add a touch of curry powder, Tabasco or paprika if you like to spice things up.

Don't be afraid to eat late...

It's not true that calories eaten after 8 pm contribute more to weight gain. What counts is how many calories you take in. If, once in a while, you do get home very late and can't face making even the simplest option for a day's dinner, don't go to bed completely empty (remember skipping meals slows metabolism). Instead, have a 50 g (2 oz) bowl of cereal with 150 ml (¼ pint) skimmed milk and a piece of fruit.

Reward yourself

Buy yourself a new perfume or aftershave. Stimulating the other senses of your body helps stop you wanting to stimulate your tastebuds with high-calorie treats.

Corn Fritters

preparation time 5 minutes **cooking time** 15 minutes **serves** 2
Kcal 155 (651 kJ) **Protein** 4 g **Carbohydrate** 21 g **Fat** 6 g

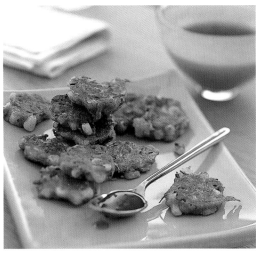

Corn Fritters

1 tablespoon olive oil
4 tablespoons frozen sweetcorn
2 tablespoons self-raising wholemeal flour
1 teaspoon vegetarian bouillon powder
2 tablespoons soya milk
1 teaspoon cider vinegar
1 dessertspoon chopped chives
¼–½ red chilli, deseeded and finely chopped (optional)
freshly ground black pepper
1 tablespoon sweet chilli sauce, to serve

1 Heat 1 teaspoon of the oil in a frying pan and fry the sweetcorn for a few minutes until hot.

2 Combine the flour, bouillon powder, milk, vinegar, chives, chilli, if using, and pepper in a bowl. Add the sweetcorn to the flour mixture and stir thoroughly.

3 Heat the remaining oil in the frying pan, then add tablespoonfuls of the corn mixture, spacing them well apart. Fry on both sides until light golden brown.

4 Transfer the fritters to a roasting tin and bake in a preheated oven, 180°C (350°F), Gas Mark 4, for 5–10 minutes until risen a little. Serve the fritters with sweet chilli sauce for dipping.

Buy fresh today

- Grapefruit (fresh or canned) and tomatoes (for breakfast option 2)
- Apple
- Avocado
- Berries (fresh or frozen)
- Spinach
- Frozen sweetcorn, cider vinegar, fresh chives and optional red chilli (or a Quorn steak)
- Vegetarian feta cheese (preferably reduced-fat)
- Soft tofu, if you don't eat eggs (for breakfast option 2)
- Pitta bread (white or wholemeal)
- Reduced-fat potato crisps
- Canned kidney beans

Today's plan

Breakfast

Option ❶ Pear Pancakes (see page 41); 150 ml (¼ pint) **skimmed milk** or **calcium-enriched soya milk**.

Option ❷ 2 **crumpets** or 2 slices of **granary or wholemeal bread**, toasted, each topped with 1 teaspoon **peanut butter** or 2 teaspoons **low-fat cream cheese**, plus 1 sliced **pear**; 150 ml (¼ pint) **skimmed milk** or **calcium-enriched soya milk**.

Mid-morning snack

3 handfuls of fresh or frozen **blackberries** (or other berries such as blueberries, strawberries, raspberries, or red or blackcurrants) served with 125 g (4 oz) pot **soya or low-fat dairy yogurt**, plus 10 **almonds.**

Lunch

200 g (7 oz) **baked potato** (see Quick tip, page 34) topped with a huge coleslaw-style salad of shredded **cabbage**, **carrot** and **onion** mixed with 2 teaspoons **low-calorie dressing**. Add 1 tablespoon **raisins** and 15 **almonds.**

Afternoon snack

15 black, green or mixed **olives**, a few **celery** sticks and 25 g (1 oz) **feta cheese**.

Dinner

Option ❶: Simple stir-fry of any **vegetables** you like with 50 g (2 oz) **tofu**, served on a bed of 50 g (2 oz) dry weight **egg noodles**. Add **sweet chilli sauce** or fresh chopped **chilli** to taste.

Option ❷: Thai Noodles with Vegetables and Tofu (see page 63).

Slow but steady...

Losing weight should be a slow and steady process so the figure on the scales is not always the best thing to focus on for motivation. Today think of five other benefits that you'll get from going on this diet (more energy, better skin, increased hydration, for example) and focus on those as well.

Reward yourself

Treat yourself by renting your favourite DVD and just enjoying a night in front of the television. Sometimes the best reward (and stress reliever) is just to do nothing.

Quick tip

We all have times in the day when we nibble; if yours is as soon as you come in from work, buy some sugar-free gum to stop you raiding the fridge while this evening's dish is marinating.

Thai Noodles with Vegetables and Tofu

preparation time 20 minutes, plus marinating **cooking time** 40 minutes **serves** 4
Kcal 276 (1160 kJ) **Protein** 18 g **Carbohydrate** 33 g **Fat** 6 g

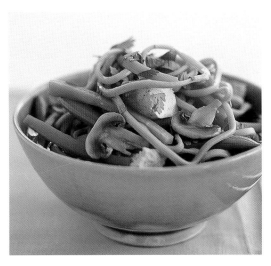

250 g (8 oz) tofu, diced

2 tablespoons dark soy sauce

1 teaspoon grated lime rind

1.8 litres (3 pints) vegetable stock

2 slices of fresh root ginger

2 garlic cloves

2 coriander sprigs

2 lemon grass stalks, crushed

1 red chilli, bruised

175 g (6 oz) dried egg noodles

125 g (4 oz) button mushrooms, sliced

2 large carrots, cut into matchsticks

125 g (4 oz) sugar snap peas

125 g (4 oz) Chinese cabbage, shredded

2 tablespoons chopped fresh coriander

Thai noodles with Vegetables and Tofu

1 Put the tofu in a shallow dish with the soy sauce and lime rind. Leave to marinate for 30 minutes.

2 Meanwhile, put the vegetable stock in a large saucepan and add the ginger, garlic, coriander sprigs, lemon grass and chilli. Bring to the boil then reduce the heat, cover and simmer for 30 minutes.

3 Strain the vegetable stock into another saucepan, return to the boil and plunge in the noodles. Add the sliced mushrooms and marinated tofu with any remaining marinade. Reduce the heat and simmer gently for 4 minutes.

4 Stir in the carrots, sugar snap peas, Chinese cabbage and chopped coriander. Cook for a further 3–4 minutes then serve.

Buy fresh today

- Pears
- Berries
- Potato
- Cabbage
- Carrots
- Onion
- Celery
- Lime
- Vegetarian feta cheese (preferably reduced-fat)
- Tofu
- Buttermilk, caster sugar and cinnamon (for breakfast option 1) or crumpets (for breakfast option 2)
- Olives
- Raisins
- Button mushrooms
- Sugar snap peas
- Chinese cabbage
- Red chillies
- Lemon grass
- Root ginger
- Fresh coriander

Today's plan

Breakfast

Option **1** Wild Mushroom Omelette (see page 65) served with 1 slice of **granary or wholemeal toast** and 150 ml (¼ pint) glass of **grapefruit juice**.

Option **2** 2 slices of **granary or wholemeal toast**, topped with 25 g (1 oz) grated **reduced-fat cheese** and 1 sliced **tomato**, then grilled. 150 ml (¼ pint) glass of **grapefruit juice**.

Mid-morning snack

2 handfuls of fresh or frozen **blackberries** (or other berries such as blueberries, strawberries, raspberries, or red or blackcurrants) mixed into 125 g (4 oz) pot **soya or low-fat dairy yogurt**.

Lunch

Salad of **baby spinach** or **watercress**, topped with 5 **sun-dried tomatoes**, 50 g (2 oz) **feta cheese** and 5 chopped **walnuts**. Add 1 tablespoon **low-calorie dressing** such as Caesar.

Afternoon snack

2 **crispbreads** or **oatcakes** topped with ¼ **avocado**, mashed, or 2 teaspoons **low-fat cream cheese**.

Dinner

Vegetarian bolognese made with 75 g (3 oz) **Quorn or soya mince** and one-third of a 500 g (1 lb) jar of ready-made **vegetarian pasta sauce** or 2 servings of **Spicy Tomato Sauce** (see page 45). Serve with 75 g (3 oz) dry weight **pasta**.

Don't let your weekend break derail you...

If you're craving the foods you had over the weekend, remind yourself that you can have them all over again next weekend if you want them. It'll also help to do something different this evening. Many of us link evening activities with certain foods – changing things even slightly can stop the cravings starting.

Reward yourself

Do a 2-minute de-stress stretch. Just take any muscle that feels tense and slowly stretch it as far as it will go – for example, clasp your hands high above your head and push your palms to the sky. Hold each move for 10–20 seconds, and slowly release. Afterwards you'll feel relaxed and energized.

Quick tip

Your lunchtime salad can easily be made in the morning before work and taken with you. Just carry the dressing separately in a small watertight pot.

Wild Mushroom Omelette

preparation time 10 minutes **cooking time** 20 minutes **serves** 4
Kcal 282 (1172 kJ) **Protein** 19 g **Carbohydrate** 0.7 g **Fat** 23 g

2 tablespoons butter or margarine
200 g (7 oz) wild mushrooms, trimmed and sliced
8 large eggs, beaten
freshly ground black pepper
2 tablespoons chopped parsley
50 g (2 oz) Gruyère cheese, grated

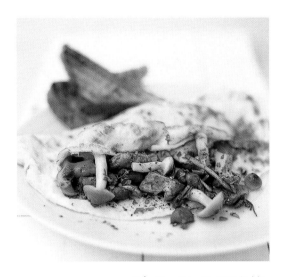

wild mushroom omelette

1 Melt a little of the butter or margarine in an omelette pan, add the mushrooms and sauté for 5–6 minutes until cooked and any moisture has evaporated. Remove the mushrooms from the pan.

2 Melt a little more butter or margarine in the same pan and add one-quarter of the beaten egg. Season well with pepper and stir with a wooden spoon, bringing the cooked egg to the centre of the pan and allowing the runny egg to flow to the edge of the pan and cook.

3 When there is only a little liquid egg left, sprinkle over a few mushrooms and some of the parsley and Gruyère. Fold the omelette over, tip on to a warm serving plate and keep warm while you make 3 more omelettes in the same way.

Buy fresh today

- Wild mushrooms, fresh parsley and vegetarian Gruyère (for breakfast option 1)
- Tomato and reduced-fat vegetarian cheese (for breakfast option 2)
- Berries (fresh or frozen)
- Baby spinach or watercress
- Avocado (if using)
- Quorn or soya mince
- Vegetarian feta cheese (preferably reduced-fat)
- Ready-made vegetarian pasta sauce (or the ingredients for the recipe on page 15)
- Sun-dried tomatoes

Today's plan

Reward yourself

Try body brushing – it invigorates your body, gives your skin a glow and flushes out the excess fluid that can add inches.

1 Get a medium-handled body brush from your local pharmacy or healthfood store and work on dry skin before taking a bath or shower.

2 Starting at your feet, brush upwards in long firm strokes, focusing first on your lower legs, then the area of your hips and thighs. Work on both the front and back of your body.

Check the noise levels around you...

Researchers at Pennsylvania State University have found that we find it harder to control ourselves around food if the levels of background noise around us are too high.

Quick tip

Always buy almonds still in their skins as these contain higher levels of antioxidants than 'blanched' almonds. Eating the almond skin increases the fibre content of your snack, helping keep you fuller for longer.

Breakfast

Smoothie made from **1 banana**, 2 handfuls of fresh or frozen **blueberries** (or other berries such as blackberries, strawberries, raspberries, or red or blackcurrants) and 150 ml (¼ pint) **skimmed milk** or **calcium-enriched soya milk**; 1 slice of **granary or wholemeal toast** topped with 1 teaspoon **peanut butter** or 2 teaspoons **low-fat cream cheese**.

Mid-morning snack

10 **almonds**.

Lunch

1 medium **pitta bread** or 1 slice of **granary or wholemeal bread** served as an 'open sandwich', filled with 2 tablespoons **reduced-fat coleslaw**, store-bought or homemade (made from shredded cabbage, carrot and onion mixed with a low-calorie dressing); 200 g (7 oz) serving of **lentil or vegetable soup** – store-bought or homemade (see page 71); 150 ml (¼ pint) glass of **grapefruit juice**.

Afternoon snack

1 **pear** and 4 **dried apricots**.

Dinner

Option **1** **Spinach, Butter Bean and Ricotta Frittata** (see page 67) served with 200 g (7 oz) **baked beans**.
Option **2** Huge salad of **spinach**, **red onion** and chopped **tomato**, topped with 1 **hard-boiled egg** (if you eat them), 3 tablespoons **canned chickpeas** and 1 tablespoon **sunflower seeds** and dressed with a blend of ½ tablespoon each of **balsamic vinegar**, **lemon juice** and **olive oil**.

Spinach, Butter Bean and Ricotta Frittata

preparation time 10 minutes **cooking time** 10 minutes **serves** 2
Kcal 417 (1748 kJ) **Protein** 32 g **Carbohydrate** 34 g **Fat** 18 g

1 teaspoon olive oil
1 onion, sliced
400 g (13 oz) can butter beans, drained and rinsed
200 g (7 oz) baby spinach leaves
4 eggs, beaten
50 g (2 oz) ricotta cheese
salt and freshly ground black pepper (optional)

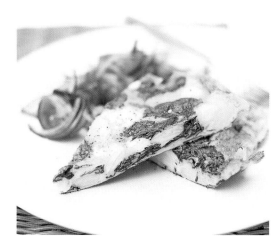

Spinach, Butter Bean and Ricotta Frittata

❶ Heat the oil in a medium frying pan, add the onion and fry for 3–4 minutes until softened. Add the butter beans and spinach and heat gently for 2–3 minutes until the spinach has wilted.

❷ Pour over the eggs, then spoon over the ricotta and season with salt and pepper, if using. Cook until almost set, then place the pan under a preheated hot grill and cook for another 1–2 minutes until golden and set.

Buy fresh today

- Banana
- Berries (fresh or frozen)
- Pear
- Onion
- Baby spinach
- Tomato (for dinner option 2)
- Vegetarian ricotta cheese (for dinner option 1)
- Reduced-fat coleslaw (or the ingredients to make your own)
- Pitta bread, white or wholemeal (if using)
- Canned butter beans and baked beans (for dinner option 1)
- Canned chickpeas (for dinner option 2)

Today's plan

Reward yourself

Book yourself a spa day – or even just a really indulgent one-off treatment like a rich body wrap, aromatherapy massage or men's facial. The more you take care of your body the more it starts to feel as if you are nurturing it. This then switches your brain into 'care' mode and it'll actually make you more inclined to make healthy eating choices – even during those weekends off.

Quick tip

You can buy ready-made bean salads from the deli counter – just drain away most of the dressing, which can be oily. Alternatively, make your own by combining 3 tablespoons canned mixed beans, or 1½ tablespoons each canned kidney beans and chickpeas with ½ tomato, chopped, 2 finely chopped coriander leaves, 2 teaspoons balsamic vinegar and 1 teaspoon olive oil.

Breakfast

Any 3 pieces/slices of **fruit** (try **watermelon**, **pear** and **banana**) served with 125 g (4 oz) pot **soya or low-fat dairy yogurt** or **fromage frais**.

Mid-morning snack

10 **almonds** and 4 **dried apricots**.

Lunch

200 g (7 oz) **baked potato** (see Quick tip, page 34) topped with 3 tablespoons **salsa** and 50 g (2 oz) grated **reduced-fat cheese**. Serve with 3 tablespoons **mixed bean salad**.

Afternoon snack

2 **oatcakes** topped with 2 tablespoons **reduced-fat hummus** or ¼ **avocado**, mashed.

Dinner

Stuffed Mushrooms (see page 69) or 2 **vegetarian sausages** served with 50 g (2 oz) dry weight **red lentils** or 200 g (7 oz) **canned lentils** and a serving of **green beans**.

Recruit a diet buddy...

Find someone who will simply listen to you for 10 minutes when you get food cravings or, even better, who will pair up with you for daily walks, runs or other activities. According to research from the University of Pittsburgh, not only are people more likely to lose weight if they diet with a buddy, but they are nearly three times more likely to keep it off.

Stuffed Mushrooms

preparation time 5 minutes **cooking time** 20–25 minutes **serves** 2
Kcal 246 (1035 kJ) **Protein** 6.6 g **Carbohydrate** 24 g **Fat** 19 g

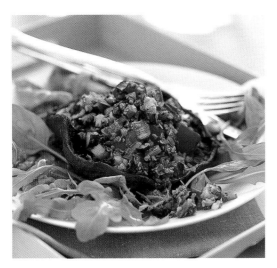

2 large, flat field mushrooms
2 tablespoons olive oil, plus extra for oiling
2 spring onions, chopped
½ red pepper, deseeded and chopped
1 small courgette, chopped
4 pitted olives, chopped
2 tablespoons porridge oats
1 tablespoon chopped basil
1 tablespoon soy sauce
1 tablespoon lime juice
salt and freshly ground black pepper

Stuffed mushrooms

❶ Wipe the mushrooms clean with damp kitchen paper, then remove the stalks and chop them.

❷ Heat the oil in a small saucepan and gently fry the chopped mushroom stalks, spring onions, red pepper, courgette, olives and oats until the oats are golden. Stir in the basil, soy sauce and lime juice.

❸ Oil the mushroom caps and place them on a baking sheet. Spoon the oat mixture on to the mushrooms, season with salt and pepper and bake in a preheated oven, 180°C (350°F), Gas Mark 4, for 15–20 minutes until the caps start to soften. Serve immediately.

Buy fresh today

- Fruits of your choice
- Potato
- Avocado or reduced-fat hummus (see Quick tip, page 58)
- mushrooms, spring onions, red pepper, courgette, lime, fresh basil and olives (or vegetarian sausages)
- Green beans
- Reduced-fat vegetarian cheese
- Bean salad

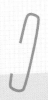

Today's plan

Breakfast

25 g (1 oz) **bran cereal** served with 150 ml (¼ pint) **skimmed milk** or **calcium-enriched soya milk** and topped with 4 chopped **dried apricots**, 6 **almonds** and 1 chopped **banana**.

Mid-morning snack

1 **pear** and 125 g (4 oz) pot **soya or low-fat dairy yogurt.**

Lunch

Option ❶ 2 slices of **granary or wholemeal toast**, each topped with 1 tablespoon **reduced-fat hummus**, served with any 400 g (13 oz) can **tomato or lentil soup**.

Option ❷ **Spicy Lentil and Tomato Soup** (see page 71) served with a large side salad of unlimited **rocket**, **celery** and **red pepper**, topped with 1 tablespoon **reduced-fat hummus.**

Afternoon snack

15 **olives** and 1 oz (25 g) **feta cheese** or a **low-fat soft cheese.**

Dinner

Couscous with Grilled Vegetables (see page 39) or 50 g (2 oz) dry weight **couscous**, topped with 200 g (7 oz) **canned ratatouille.**

Brush your teeth after eating...

Taking away the taste of food straight after eating tells your brain that the mealtime is over and stops you thinking about going back for second helpings.

Reward yourself

Splash out on a new CD. Choose something relaxing if you've had a hard week or go for something energetic if you want to boost your diet results – 45 minutes dancing or marching to music will burn up about 300 calories.

Quick tip

This soup can be made the night before and stored in the fridge. Alternatively, make up a large batch then freeze it in individual pots. You can then take one with you to work, for example, and warm it up for about 2 minutes in the microwave. The salad travels well, too – wrap the hummus in a little foil to keep it separate until just before serving.

Spicy Lentil and Tomato Soup

preparation time 20 minutes **cooking time** 40–50 minutes **serves** 4
Kcal 288 (1210 kJ) **Protein** 18 g **Carbohydrate** 28 g **Fat** 2 g

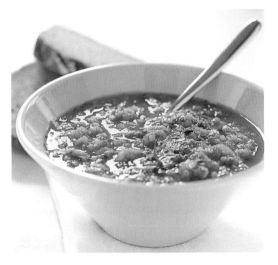

Spicy Lentil and Tomato Soup

1 tablespoon vegetable oil
1 large onion, finely chopped
2 garlic cloves, finely chopped
1 small green chilli, deseeded and finely chopped
250 g (8 oz) red lentils, washed and drained
1 bay leaf
3 celery sticks, thinly sliced
3 carrots, thinly sliced
1 leek, thinly sliced
1.5 litres (2½ pints) vegetable stock
400 g (13 oz) can chopped tomatoes
2 tablespoons tomato purée
½ tablespoon ground turmeric
½ teaspoon ground ginger
1 tablespoon fresh coriander
freshly ground black pepper
soya or low-fat dairy natural yogurt, to serve (optional)

1 Heat the oil in a large saucepan, add the onion, garlic and chilli and fry gently for 4–5 minutes until soft.

2 Add the lentils, bay leaf, celery, carrots, leek and vegetable stock. Cover and bring to the boil, then reduce the heat and simmer for 30–40 minutes. Remove the bay leaf.

3 Stir in the canned tomatoes, tomato purée, turmeric, ginger, coriander and pepper to taste. Allow to cool slightly then transfer to a food processor or blender. Process until smooth, adding more stock or water if necessary.

4 Reheat gently, before serving with a swirl of yogurt, if using.

Buy fresh today

- Banana
- Pear
- Onion, green chilli, celery, carrots, leek, fresh coriander, rocket and red pepper (for lunch option 2)
- Red and orange pepper, baby courgettes, red onions, cherry tomatoes, asparagus, lemon and fresh herbs (or canned ratatouille)
- Vegetarian feta cheese (preferably reduced-fat) or a low-fat soft cheese
- Reduced-fat hummus (see Quick tip, page 58)
- Olives
- Tomato purée, bay leaf, ground turmeric and ground ginger (for lunch option 2)

Today's plan

Reward yourself

Flick through some holiday brochures. You
don't need to book a trip, just dream – but
in that dream see yourself looking great on
the beach. Keep returning to that image,
and it'll help keep you focused on your diet.

Test your weight...

Visit your local gym or sports store
and pick up a 1 kg (2 lb) dumbbell. That's
the minimum amount of weight you should
have lost on the plan so far. It might not
seem much on the scales, but it's certainly
not light in reality – try carrying it about
for a few minutes and see.

Quick tip

Vegetarian cheeses are
now available in all sorts
of varieties including blue
varieties like the
one used in today's
risotto. This is good diet
news, as you only need a
little of strong cheeses
like this which reduces
calories.

Breakfast

Porridge made from 50 g (2 oz) porridge oats mixed as
per the instructions with a little water. Add 1 chopped
banana and serve with ½ **grapefruit** or 6 **canned
grapefruit segments**.

Mid-morning snack

6 chopped **dried apricots** mixed into 50 g (2 oz) **low-fat
cottage cheese**.

Lunch

2 'open sandwiches' made with 2 slices of **granary
or wholemeal bread** (ideally toasted) topped with ½
avocado, mashed, and sprinkled with 2 teaspoons
pumpkin seeds, ¼ **red chilli**, finely chopped, (optional)
and **lemon juice**. Serve with sticks of **carrot**, **celery** and
cucumber, plus 3 tablespoons **reduced-fat hummus**.

Afternoon snack

1 **pear**, chopped and dipped in 1 teaspoon **peanut
butter** or 25 g (1 oz) **low-fat cottage cheese**.

Dinner

Option ❶ **Green Risotto** (see page 73) served with
a green salad of **lettuce**, **celery** and **cucumber**.
Option ❷ 50 g (2 oz) dry weight **pasta** topped with
2 tablespoons **pesto** or any ready-made **vegetarian
cheese sauce**. Serve with a large side salad of **spinach**,
rocket or **watercress** and **celery**.

Green Risotto

preparation time 10 minutes   **cooking time** 25 minutes   **serves** 6

Kcal 395 (1660 kJ)   **Protein** 14 g   **Carbohydrate** 40 g   **Fat** 20 g

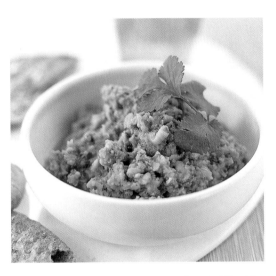

Green Risotto

1 tablespoon butter or margarine

3 garlic cloves, chopped

1 litre (1¾ pints) vegetable stock

250 g (8 oz) Arborio rice

75 ml (3 fl oz) single cream

250 g (8 oz) green beans, blanched and cut into bite-sized pieces

250 g (8 oz) asparagus, blanched and cut into bite-sized pieces

125 g (4 oz) vegetarian blue cheese

4–6 tablespoons coarsely grated vegetarian Parmesan

15 g (½ oz) basil, coarsely chopped

salt and freshly ground black pepper

1 Put the butter or margarine in a heavy-based pan, add the garlic and cook over a medium heat until golden. Meanwhile, heat the stock.

2 Add the rice to the pan containing the garlic and toss together to coat the grains in the butter or margarine.

3 Stir and add 125 ml (4 fl oz) of the hot stock to the the rice. Stir until it has been absorbed – about 5 minutes – then add another 125 ml (4 fl oz). Repeat until the rice is nearly tender.

4 Add the cream, beans and asparagus. Continue cooking until the rice is *al dente*, then stir in the blue cheese, Parmesan and basil. Season with salt and pepper and serve.

Buy fresh today

- Banana
- Grapefruit (fresh or canned)
- Green beans, asparagus, fresh basil and lettuce (for dinner option 1)
- Spinach and rocket or watercress (for dinner option 2)
- Red chilli (if using)
- Vegetarian blue cheese and vegetarian Parmesan plus single cream (for dinner option 1)
- Avocado
- Carrot
- Celery
- Cucumber
- Pear
- Low-fat cottage cheese
- Reduced-fat hummus (see Quick tip, page 58)
- Pesto (preferably reduced-fat) or ready-made vegetarian cheese sauce (for dinner option 2)
- Arborio rice (for dinner option 1)

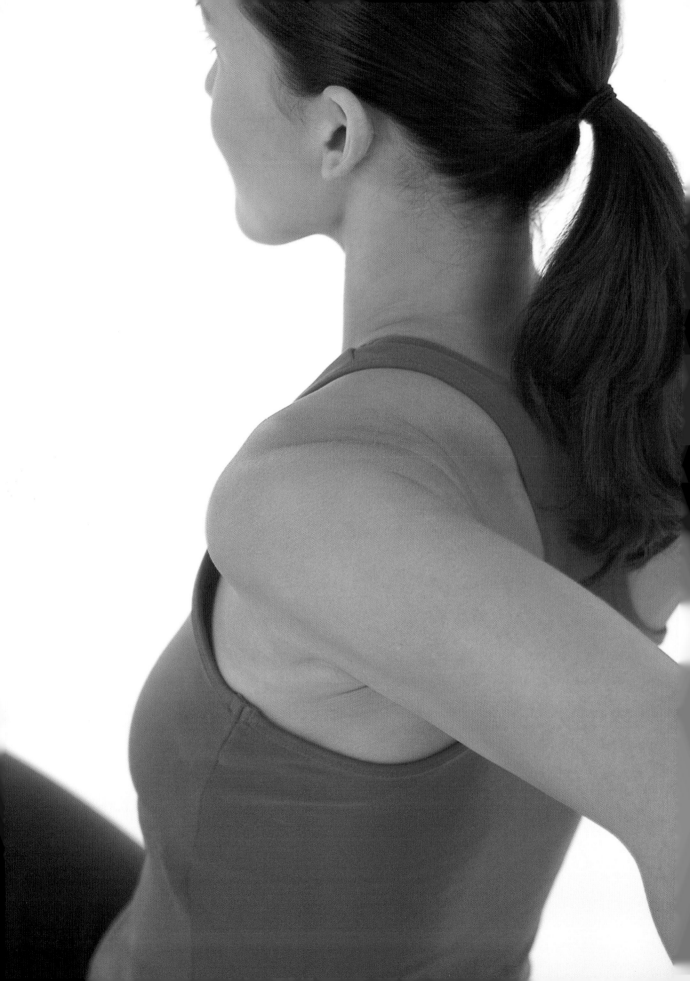

the exercise week

What you eat during the week is a major determinant of how much weight you lose, but exercise is the way to really fire things up. By burning more calories each day you increase that all-important energy deficit and get your metabolism working overtime. As a result you can increase your weight loss by another 0.5–1 kg (1–2 lb) a week.

Don't be afraid of exercise, even if you don't work out already. The types of exercise you need to do to boost metabolism and burn calories can fit into anyone's life and suit any level of fitness. Whether you're a full-time mum with kids in tow, a 40-something executive too embarrassed to put on trainers or a 20-something dynamo who can never find enough hours in the day to get things done, this plan can work for you.

Introduction

The exercise part of the diet plan is twofold. Each weekday you do a set of simple toning exercises that use your own body weight – and eventually some hand-held weights – to strengthen and tone your muscles. In addition, you do 10,000 steps (see page 100) every day to boost calorie burning. Together, these two exercise routines really maximize your weight loss results.

Using the toning plans

There are five toning plans in all, each day of the week focusing on a different type of exercise or part of your body. The reason for this is simple. Our bodies are incredibly adaptable and if you do the same workout day in, day out, within as little as six weeks you will stop getting results. By chopping and changing workouts, however, you prevent this problem and keep things challenging for your body.

Breathing correctly

Never hold your breath during toning work, just keep breathing as normally as possible throughout the whole exercise.

Some of the advanced moves require you to lift dumbbells. These are hand-held weights, which are readily available from sports and department stores and are relatively inexpensive. It is far preferable to get yourself the right equipment rather than use homemade alternatives like cans of food or bottles of water – you cannot grip and lift these in the same way so you could end up working certain muscles in the wrong way and straining yourself.

Warming up

With any exercise programme it's important that the muscles are warmed up and supple before you start. If you skip this simple step you dramatically increase your chance of injury. All it takes is at least 5 minutes' walking around the room or outside before you start your workout proper. Start off slowly, then move up to a brisker pace, pumping your arms back and forth and getting your heart rate slightly elevated.

Each exercise has a basic move and an advanced move. Everyone should start with the basics and, once these start to feel easy, move up to the advanced plan to keep things progressing. Of course every rule has an exception, and if you have never ever exercised before this applies to you. In your case, it's safer to repeat Monday's toning plan every day, or every other day, for the first four to six weeks before introducing the other workouts. This will get your body used to gentle movement and will prevent any of the stiffness and soreness that you might experience with the other routines (which work the same muscles in four to five different ways in one workout). Once you start to become fitter you can progress to the other plans.

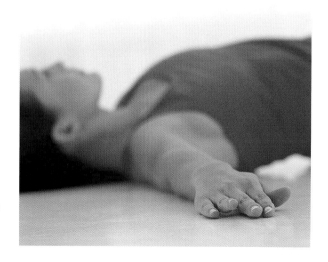

Cooling down

After any workout, you should cool down by doing stretching exercises to help release the lactic acids that can lead to muscle soreness. Use the following stretch plan daily.

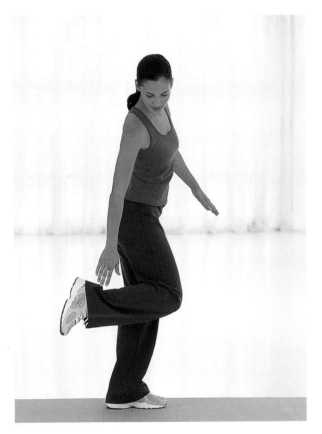 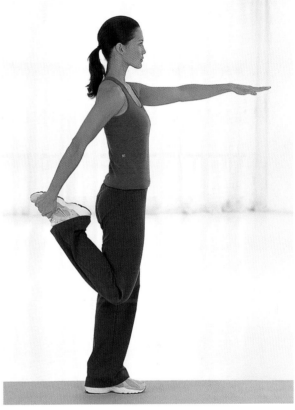

Thigh stretch

❶ Stand up straight, bend your right leg behind you and grasp your foot gently at the ankle with your right hand. Make sure you're balanced, then pull it slowly towards your bottom, trying to get it close enough so your heel just grazes your buttock. As you do so, raise your left arm horizontally in front of you.

❷ Hold this position for 30 seconds. If you want to extend the stretch further during this time, gently push your hipbone forward a little until you feel the muscle extend. Now release and repeat with the other leg.

Hamstring stretch

❶ Stand in front of a stair or low chair and place one foot on it. You should be in a position that means this elevated leg is straight, but not so extended that the knee locks. Also remember this rule on the other leg: keep your knee slightly soft. Raise your arms above your head.

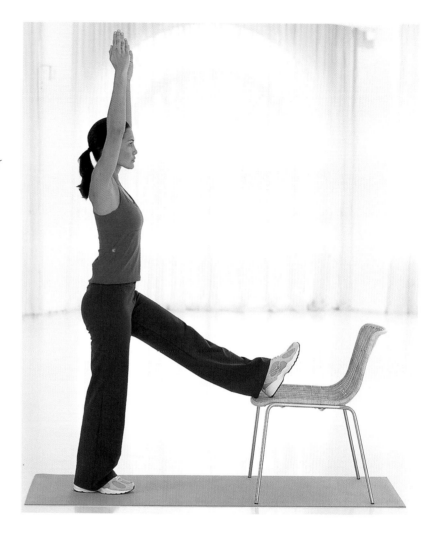

❷ If you can, rest your hands on either side of your foot. Now bend forward slightly from the waist until your feel a pull in the back of your upper thigh.

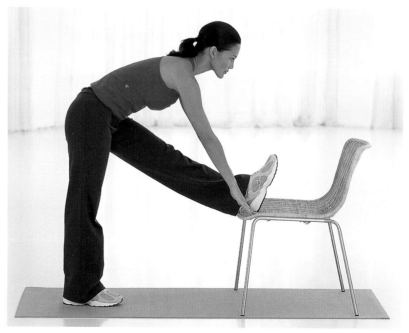

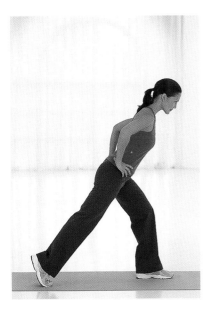
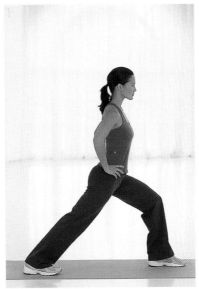

Calf stretch

❶ Stand up straight with hands on hips, then step forward with your left leg and bend your knee. As you do this your right leg will straighten and the heel will come off the floor.

❷ Keeping your left leg where it is, gently try and push the heel of your right leg back down about 2.5 cm (1 in). Hold for 20–30 seconds, then release and repeat with the other leg.

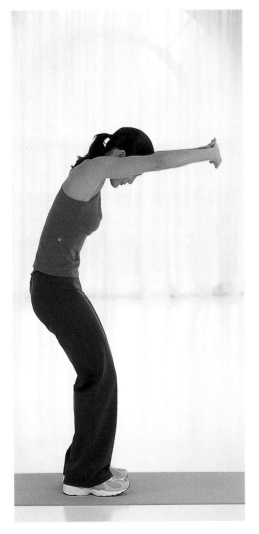
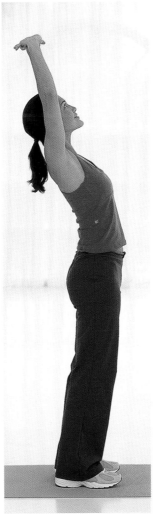

Upper body stretch

❶ Stand up straight with your arms by your sides. Now link your fingers and turn your palms outwards, straightening your arms out in front of you. Bend your body slightly from the hips and hold for 30 seconds then release.

❷ With your fingers still linked, push your arms up above your head. Hold for 30 seconds then release.

Today's workout tones and strengthens the whole body, giving you a great introduction to your exercise week and helping you create a healthy, balanced shape from top to toe.

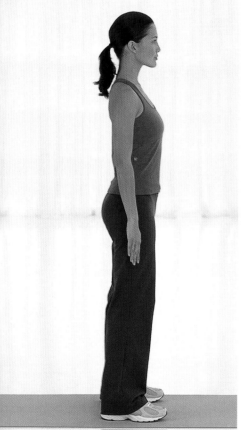

whole body

Squats

❶ Stand up straight with your feet hip width apart.

❷ Squat down as if you were going to sit. As you lower yourself, bring your arms out horizontally in front of you.

❸ Use your thigh and buttock muscles to push yourself back up to a standing position. Perform three sets of 10–20 squats.

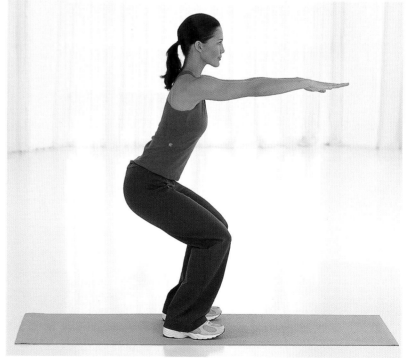

Advanced move

Perform the squats as above but hold a 2-5 kg (4-11 lb) dumbbell in each hand and hang your arms by your sides to make your thigh and buttock muscles work harder.

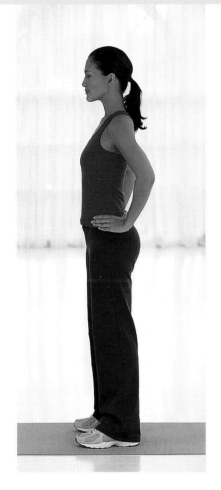

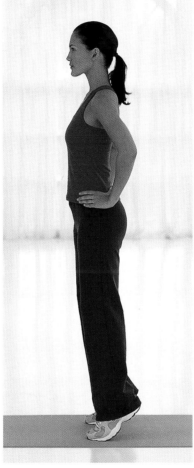

Calf raises

❶ Stand up straight with your legs together and your hands on your hips.

❷ Lift yourself up on to your toes, hold for 1 second then lower. Repeat 10 times. Change the position of your feet so that your heels are together but your toes point outwards. As before, lift yourself up again then lower. Repeat 10 times.

❸ Change position again so your toes are together but your heels are apart. Lift and lower as before and repeat 10 times.

Advanced move

Repeat each move as above, but after the tenth repetition, pause and do a tiny little pulsing move, pushing up and down quickly 10 times.

Simple curl-ups

1 Lie on your back with your knees bent and your arms behind your head to support its weight. Contract your tummy muscles as if trying to press your navel against your spine.

2 Keeping your tummy muscles taut and breathing normally throughout, gently curl up just high enough for your shoulder blades to leave the floor.

3 Lower yourself slowly back down. Perform three sets of 10 curl-ups.

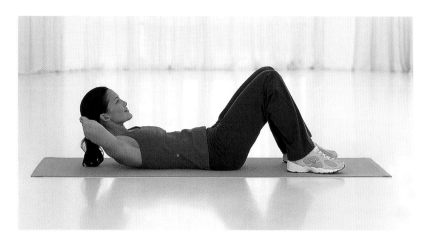

Advanced move

Repeat the move above, but at the top of the tenth lift gently pulse up and down about 2.5 cm (1 in) higher, 5–10 times.

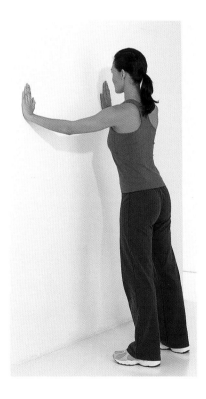

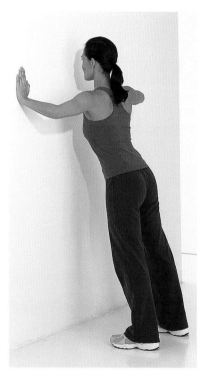

Easy press-ups

1 Stand, facing a wall, about 15 cm (6 in) away from it.

2 Lean forward, bend your arms and place your hands on the wall, slightly more than shoulder width apart. Contract your tummy muscles and try to keep them taut throughout the move, while all the time breathing normally.

3 Using your back and shoulder muscles, gently push yourself backwards away from the wall so your arms almost straighten. Then slowly lower yourself back to the leaning forward starting position. Repeat 10–20 times.

Advanced move

Move your press-up to the floor. Start by kneeling on all fours, with your hands flat on the floor, slightly more than shoulder width apart. Push your upper body forward so that your weight is supported by your knees and hands. Gently lower yourself down by bending your arms. Lift your ankles off the floor and cross them in the air. Build up to three sets of 10 press-ups.

Simple shoulder lifts

❶ Stand up straight with your feet hip width apart. Raise your arms to your sides to shoulder height, then bend your arms so that your hands are at chin height and curl them into tight fists.

❷ Raising from the shoulders, straighten your arms above your head to the point just before your elbows lock and bring your fists together.

❸ Lower and repeat 10–20 times.

At the gym

If you prefer to go to the gym to do your workouts, the following circuit will give the same results as the five Monday exercises.

- **Leg press:** do three sets of 12, pushing with your feet flat.
- **Leg press:** do three sets of 12, pushing with your toes.
- **Ab roller (standard position):** do three sets of 12.
- **Lat pulldown:** do three sets of 12.
- **Shoulder press:** do three sets of 12.

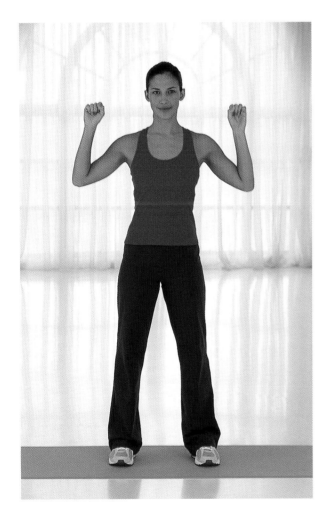

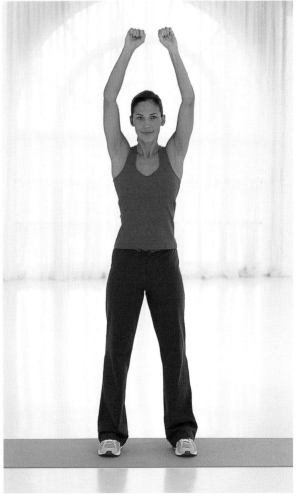

Advanced move

Do the same move but with a 2–5 kg (4–11 lb) dumbbell in each hand.

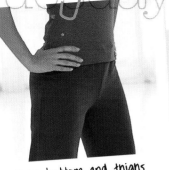

legs, bottom and thighs

Today's circuit tones the legs, bottom and thighs, which are problem areas for many women. The good news is that because these are large muscles they tone up quickly, creating a more streamlined shape fast.

Wide squats

1 Stand up straight with hands on hips, your legs wide apart and your knees turned out to a 45° angle.

2 Squat down as if you were going to sit, but make sure your knees don't extend further forward than your ankles. Focus on lowering your bottom, not widening your legs further. Hold for 1–2 seconds.

3 Use your buttock and thigh muscles to push yourself back up to the starting position. Repeat 10–15 times. Relax then do two more sets.

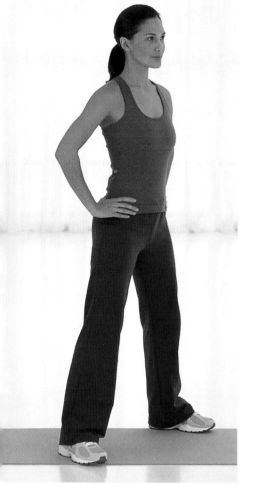

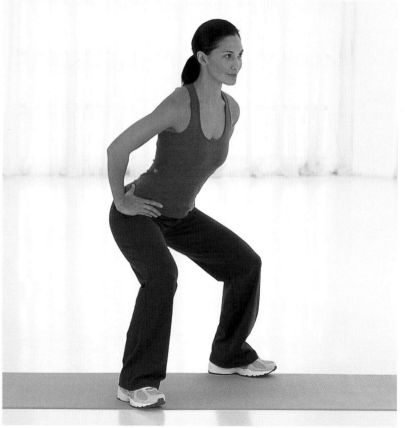

Advanced move

Perform the squats as above but hold a 2–5 kg (4–11 lb) dumbbell in each hand and hang your arms by your side to make your thigh and buttock muscles work harder.

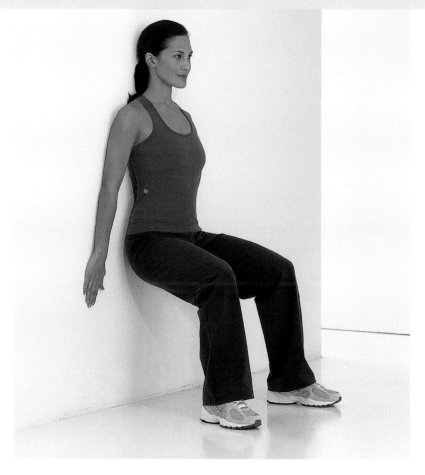

Wall squats

❶ Stand with your back resting against a wall.

❷ Bending your legs, gently slide down the wall as if you were going to sit, but you are supported by your legs instead of a seat. Be careful as you do this that your knees go no further forward than your ankles.

❸ Keeping your back flat against the wall, hover in this position for up to 1 minute.

Advanced move

Repeat the move up to 5 times. If this gets too easy, repeat the move holding a 2-5 kg (4-11 lb) dumbbell in each hand, resting them on your thighs as you hover.

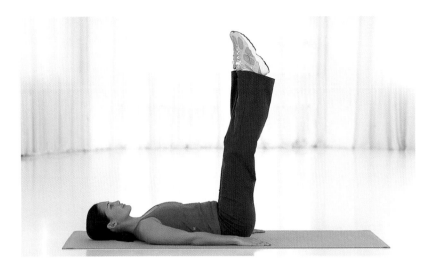

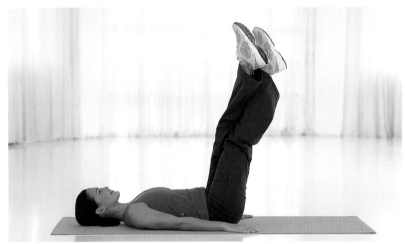

Scissor legs

❶ Lie on your back, contract your tummy muscles and press your lower back firmly into the floor. With your legs together, bend your knees, then point your legs to the ceiling as straight as you can get them.

❷ Open your legs, taking them to the sides, then bring them back together, crossing your ankles slightly. Now open them again.

❸ Repeat this scissor action fairly quickly 10–20 times, crossing alternate ankles in front of each other. Throughout the exercise, keep your tummy muscles taut, your breathing normal and your back pushed firmly into the floor.

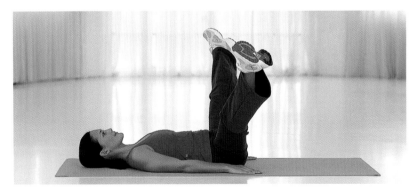

Advanced move

Repeat as above, but at the end of your repetitions keep your legs close together and cross your ankles over using small quick movements 10–20 times. Keep your back flat against the floor and your tummy muscles taut throughout.

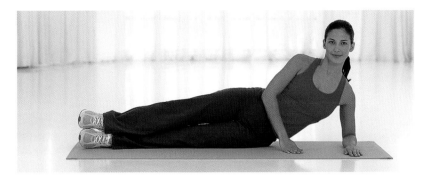

Abductors

❶ Lie on your side with one leg on top of the other and your hips facing forwards. Support your upper body with your forearm flat on the floor.

❷ Slowly raise the top leg, then lower it back down.

❸ Repeat 10–20 times, then turn on to your other side and repeat the action with the other leg uppermost.

Advanced move

Repeat the move above, but at the top of your tenth repetition, gently pulse your foot up and down about 2.5 cm (1 in) higher, 20–30 times.

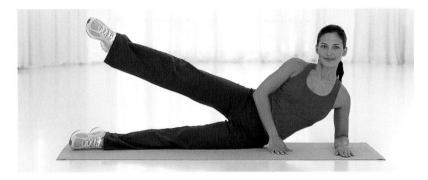

Adductors

❶ Take up the same starting position as above, then bend the top leg and place your foot in front of the lower leg, at a 90° angle to it.

❷ Slowly lift the lower leg 5–8 cm (2–3 in) off the floor. Hold for 1 second then lower it.

❸ Perform three sets of 20, then lie on your other side and repeat the action with the other leg.

Advanced move

Repeat as above, but at the top of your tenth repetition, gently pulse your foot up and down about 2.5 cm (1 in) higher, 10–20 times.

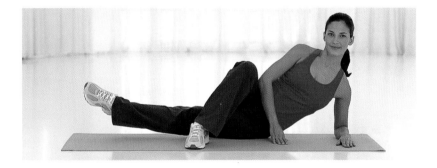

At the gym

As before, you can adapt some of Tuesday's five exercises to do at the gym.

- **Leg press:** do three sets of 12, pushing with your feet flat.
- **Wall squats:** Do the squats as on page 85, but make it harder by putting a stability ball between your back and the wall.
- **Scissor legs:** Do the scissor legs as directed left, or get a small stability ball, lie on the floor and put the ball between your feet. Gently squeeze the ball 20–30 times.
- **Abductor/adductor:** do three sets of 12 on each machine.

the exercise week **87**

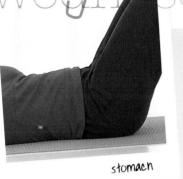

stomach

Today's exercises help create a flatter, firmer stomach and also increase the stability of the 'core' muscles – the ones that we need for good posture and a strong, healthy back.

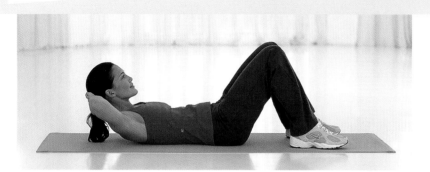

Simple curl-ups

① Lie on your back with your knees bent and your arms behind your head to support its weight. Contract your tummy muscles as if trying to push your navel against your spine.

② Gently lift up as if you were doing a sit-up, but as you lift up, twist from the waist to the right as if your left elbow were going over to touch your right knee. Hold for a second, lower yourself back down until just before your left shoulder touches the floor, then repeat this move 10 times on this side.

③ Lower completely back down to the starting position, then repeat the move as if your right elbow were going to meet your left knee.

Advanced move

Repeat the move above, but at the top of the tenth lift gently pulse up and down about 2.5 cm (1 in) higher, 5–10 times.

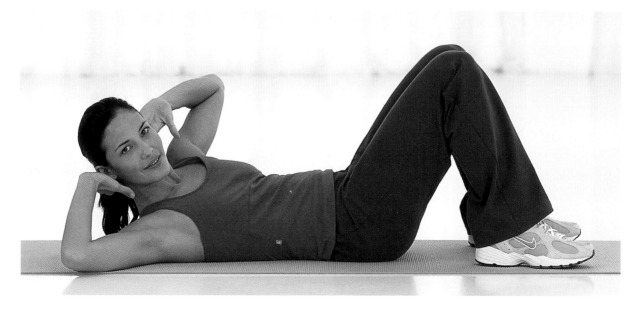

Bridges

❶ Lie on your back with your knees bent and your arms by your sides. Contract your tummy muscles as if trying to press your navel against your spine.

❷ Tilt your pelvis forward so your bottom lifts slightly off the ground.

❸ Now, very slowly and working from the bottom of your spine, curl it up and off the floor, vertebra by vertebra, until you reach your shoulder blades.

❹ Slowly roll back down, again aiming to move vertebra by vertebra. Make sure you're not holding your breath – you should be breathing normally throughout. Repeat the complete movement 3 times.

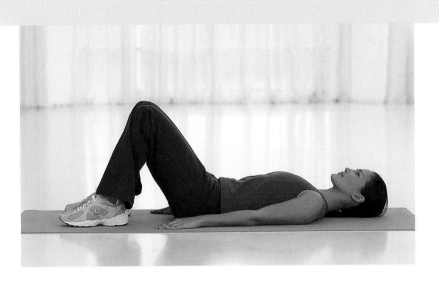

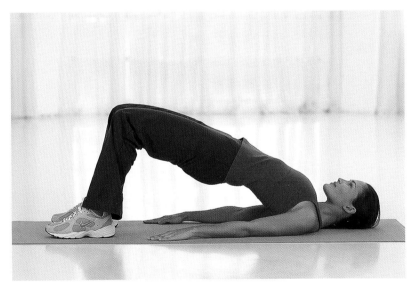

Advanced move

Repeat 5 times, but aim to be even slower and more controlled each time.

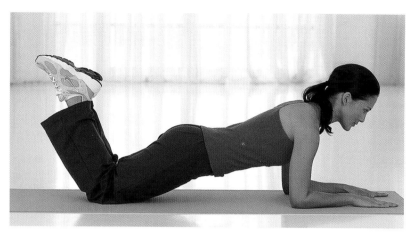

Simple planks

❶ Kneel on all fours, with your hands flat on the floor. Lower your upper body forward so that your forearms lie along the floor and your weight is supported by your elbows/forearms and knees.Raise your feet off the floor.

❷ Contract your tummy muscles as if trying to press your navel against your spine. Keep breathing steadily and hold this position for up to 1 minute. Release and repeat 5 times.

Advanced move

Hold the above position for 2 minutes each time, or try straightening your legs so that your weight is supported by your elbows/forearms and toes.

Knee drops

❶ Lie on your back with your feet off the floor and your knees bent at a 90° angle to your thighs, so that your shins are parallel to the floor. Stretch your arms out to the sides in line with your shoulders.

❷ Contract your tummy muscles and make sure you breathe normally throughout. Moving your lower body but keeping your shoulder blades still, move both your knees over to the right and lower them 5–8 cm (2–3 in) towards the floor.

❸ Bring your knees back up using your tummy muscles. Do this 5 times, then repeat on your left side.

Advanced move

Keeping both shoulder blades still on the floor, aim to twist far enough round that you actually touch the floor with the outer knee.

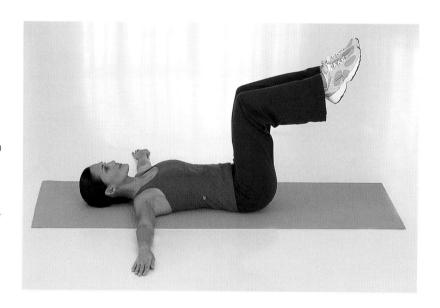

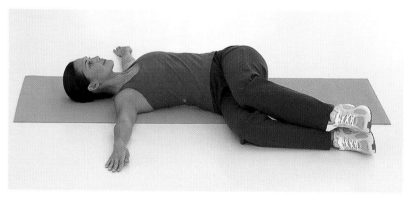

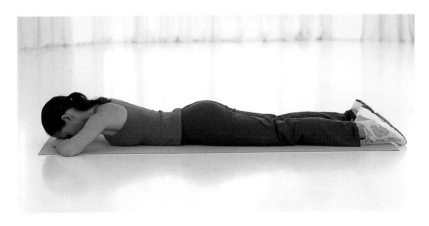

Lower back strengtheners

❶ Lie on your front with your elbows bent and your forehead resting on the backs of your hands.

❷ Contract your tummy muscles as before then, breathing normally throughout, slowly lift your head, neck and shoulders off the floor.

❸ Lower slowly back down and repeat 10 times.

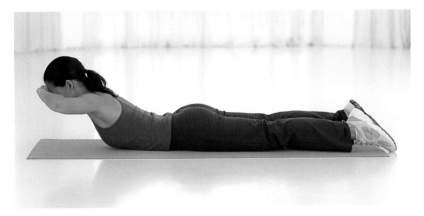

Advanced move

Repeat the move as above. At the top of the raise, move your elbows out to the sides and down your body to your waist. You'll feel your shoulder blades move down your back. Move back up to the start and repeat 5-10 times.

At the gym

Abdominal muscles are best worked without the help of exercise machines, so at the gym you should repeat the above exercises as directed, or ask an instructor how to adapt them with a stability ball. The ball makes you work slightly off balance so that you involve more 'core' muscles in your workout.

arms, back and shoulders

Today you will be working your arms, back and shoulders so as to create a lean upper body – women in particular will appreciate creating toned arms that are spaghetti-strap gorgeous!

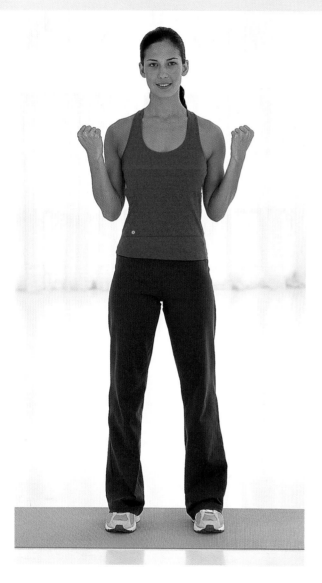

Bicep curls

❶ Stand up straight with your arms by your sides, palms facing forward. Lightly clench your fists.

❷ With your upper arms held closely to your sides, curl up your arms to bring your fists towards your shoulders, really focusing on contracting the bicep muscle at the top of each arm and rolling it through the move.

❸ When your fists reach your shoulders, lower them back down. Repeat 15–20 times.

Advanced move

Hold a 2-5 kg (4-11 lb) dumbbell in each hand and repeat. Remember that it's the contracting and rolling part of the move that is most important, otherwise you're just working your forearms.

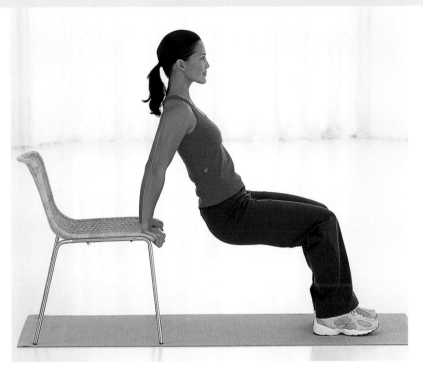

Tricep dips

❶ Sitting on the edge of a sturdy chair with your feet well forward, flat on the floor, place your hands either side of your hips and grasp the edge of the seat. Keeping your upper body straight, lower yourself off the chair so that you are supported by your bent arms.

❷ Use your arms to raise and lower yourself about 15–20 cm (6–8 in), keeping your hips close to the chair. Do three sets of 10 dips.

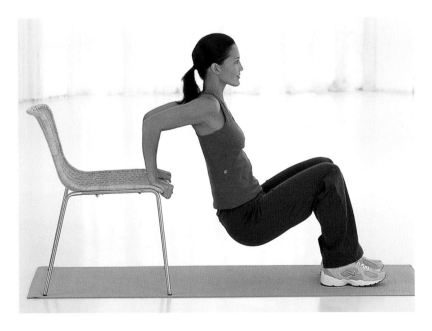

Advanced move

Repeat as above but as you move up and down, lift one leg slightly off the floor so that your weight is supported by one leg only.

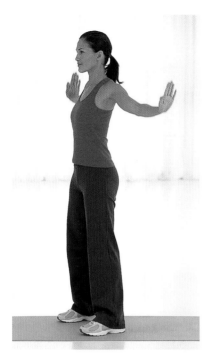
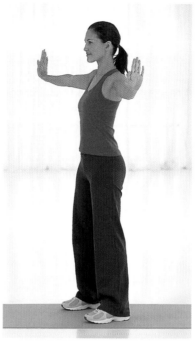

Arm circles

❶ Stand up straight with your feet hip width apart and your arms outstretched to the sides at shoulder height. Bend your hands at the wrists so that they are at 90° to your forearms.

❷ Move the wrists and palms of your hands in tiny clockwise circles, while you count to 10. (Although the tiny circles are powered by your palms and wrists the whole of your arms actually move from the shoulder down.)

❸ Now repeat the movement, anti-clockwise, while you count to 10.

❹ Relax your arms, and repeat the sequence 4 times.

Advanced move

Lengthen the exercise by counting to 20, then to 30. Once this too becomes easy you can make the circles with your arms progressively bigger.

Simple chest press

❶ Stand up straight, feet hip width apart. Lift your arms parallel to your shoulders, forearms pointing towards the ceiling, hands clasped in a light fist (visually this is very similar to the starting position to the simple shoulder raises on page 83).

❷ Moving from the shoulder, so your whole arm moves 'as one', bring your arms together so your forearms press against each other. As you do this, clench the muscles in your chest/under your breasts and focus on stretching the muscles across your shoulder blades.

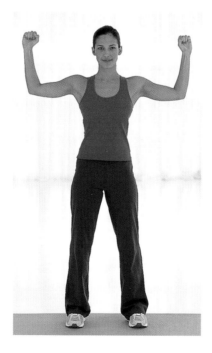
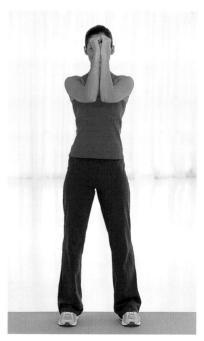

Advanced move

Repeat the move holding a 2–5kg (4–11 lb) dumbbell in each hand.

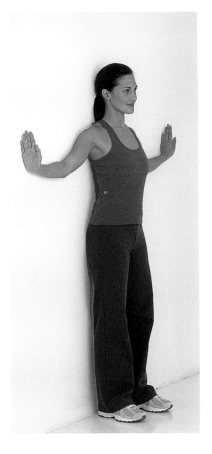
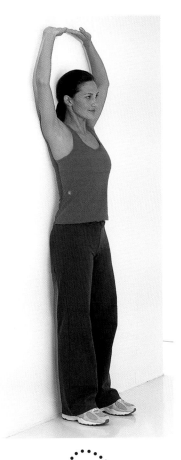
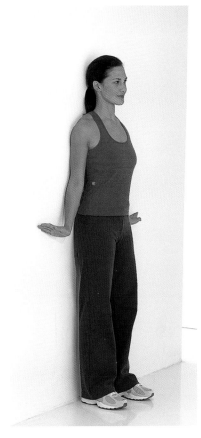

Wall angels

1 Stand up straight with your hips, your back and your arms, outstretched to the sides at shoulder height, against a wall. Bend your elbows, pointing your fingers towards the ceiling.

2 Slowly move your arms up overhead until your fingers touch, then bring them far enough down so that your elbows touch your waist, keeping your hand at 90° to your arms.

3 Repeat the move, performing three sets of 10.

At the gym

As always, you can do the day's toning exercises using machines at the gym if you prefer.

- **Bicep curl:** do three sets of 12.
- **Tricep extension:** do three sets of 12.
- **Arm circles:** Do the circles as on page 94 or, to make it harder, use a resistance band. Hold one end of the band between your thumb and forefinger, stand on the other and perform the exercise.
- **Shoulder press:** do three sets of 12.
- **Lat pulldown:** do three sets of 12.

Advanced move

Repeat the exercise but with a 2–5 kg (4–11 lb) dumbbell in each hand.

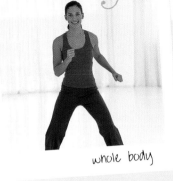

whole body

Today you'll work the whole body with more aerobic types of toning moves. To make these exercises harder, try to increase the number of movements you perform in the time specified.

Rapid knee lifts

❶ Stand up straight with your feet together then start marching on the spot, raising your knees high. Aim to work hard enough so that you can still speak but not carry on a conversation.

❷ Continue marching for 1 minute.

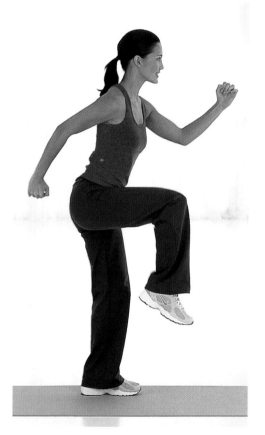

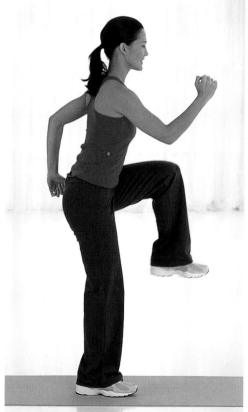

Advanced move
Speed up to increase the number of knee lifts you perform in the 1 minute.

Side steps

1 Stand up straight with your feet together.

2 Take a large step to the side with your left leg, then a large step to the right-hand side with your right leg.

3 Bring your left leg back in, followed by your right leg.

4 Keep repeating this movement for 1 minute, aiming to do as many steps as you can.

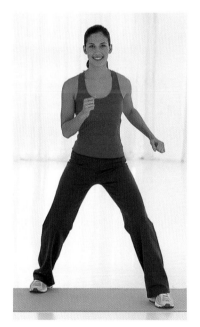 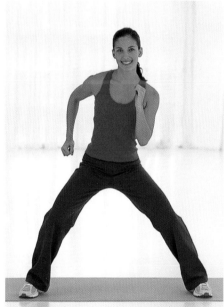 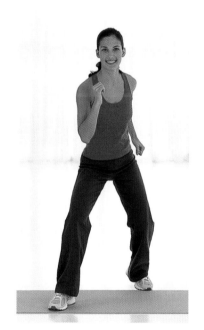

Advanced move
Speed up to increase the number of sideways steps you perform in the 1 minute.

Stair climbs

❶ This exercise simply involves climbing up and down stairs for 2 minutes. Go as fast as you can while sticking to the 'still being able to speak' rule (see page 96).

❷ If you really are new to exercise, skip the stair part of this move for a few weeks. Focus instead on simply walking briskly around the room for 2 minutes.

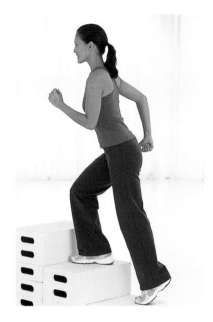
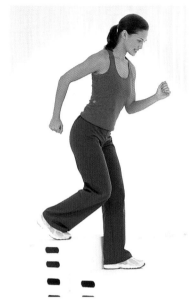

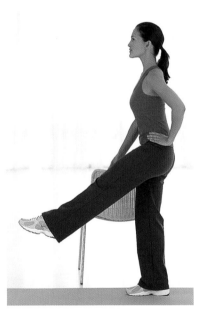
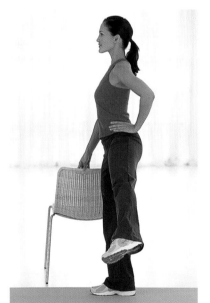
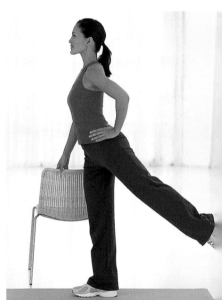

Leg kicks

❶ Stand up straight, side on to a chair or wall, holding it lightly with your right hand for balance. Contract your tummy muscles.

❷ Keeping it as straight as possible, kick your left leg out in front of you to the point just before your knee locks. Still keeping it

straight and without touching the floor, take it out to the left and slightly back – you'll end up roughly parallel to your right leg. Still keeping it straight and in the air, bring the leg further back and in to the right, so you end up with it extended straight out behind you. Now bring it back to the starting point. The whole move

feels like drawing a triangle with your foot.

❸ Repeat for 30 seconds then swap legs. Make sure you breathe steadily and keep the kicks controlled – you don't want to feel your knee snapping back and forth. If your leg feels out of control, slow down.

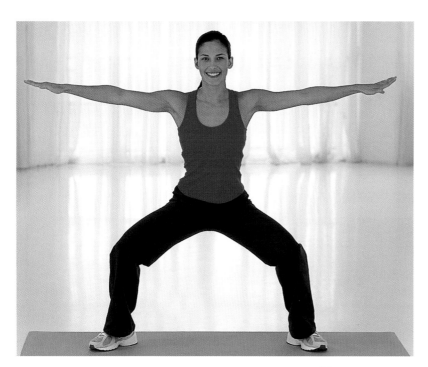

Jumping jacks

❶ Stand up straight with your feet together and your arms down by your sides.

❷ Bend your knees and then jump up in the air. As you do so, widen your legs and raise your arms to shoulder height.

❸ Land with your legs wide apart, then jump again, reversing the move so you end up with your arms by your sides and your feet back together again.

❹ Repeat for 1 minute.

Note: If you haven't exercised before, or if you weigh more than about 6 kg (14 lb) over your recommended weight, don't do this exercise yet. Do half-jacks instead until you become fitter and you lose a bit more weight. From the same starting position described above, take a big step sideways to the right with your right leg as you raise both arms up above your head. Then bring your leg back in again as you lower your arms. Repeat this 10 times with your right leg, then swap to your left leg.

At the gym

This is an aerobic circuit programme, which is so short you'd be unlikely to go specifically to the gym to do it. However, if you want to do a workout at the gym today, spend 2–5 minutes on each of the following exercise machines, working at an intensity level of 6–8 out of 10 (depending on your level of fitness and the time available):

- **Treadmill**
- **Rowing machine**
- **Stepper**
- **Cross-trainer**
- **Grinder** – this looks like a big cycle wheel but is operated by your arms. If your gym doesn't have one, do another session on the rowing machine instead.

Burning extra calories

The daily toning exercises on the previous pages help rev your metabolism indirectly by increasing muscle mass, but they burn only 50–100 calories a session – depending on your body weight and workout intensity. This helps with your daily calorie deficit, but to increase your 0.5 kg (1 lb) weight loss a week to 1 kg (2 lb) or more, take 10,000 steps every day.

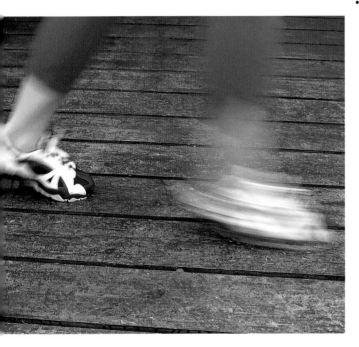

What if I prefer to exercise in the gym?

Then that's fantastic, keep it up. Any extra calories you burn through gym work or playing sport will increase your calorie deficit and maximize your results, but do try to increase the amount of 'stealth' work you do each day as well. If you can add 10,000 steps a day to your normal workout, you'll be burning off an excess of 3,000 calories every five days – and definitely achieving that 1 kg (2 lb) a week weight loss.

The 10,000 steps plan

This simply involves aiming to increase the number of steps you take each day, be it at home, at work or out and about (see box opposite), to at least 10,000 (the average office worker currently does about 2,000). Ten thousand steps equate to about 8 km (5 miles) and will give you a calorie burn per day of around 500. You simply measure the number of steps you walk with an inexpensive device called a pedometer (widely available in sports and department stores), which you clip on to your waistband each morning.

Do not try to do your 10,000 steps wearing uncomfortable shoes as it will only end in pain. If you have to wear smart or high-heeled shoes to work, keep a pair of trainers or other practical shoes handy and focus on stepping at lunchtime. Remember that speed doesn't matter. Walking faster does not give you extra step benefits so if you find it hard to walk fast, then it's fine to keep it slow.

Getting started

If you live a very sedentary life – you can't walk for more than 5 minutes without experiencing pain or becoming short of breath – don't aim for the 10,000 steps all in one go. Instead, spend your first day wearing the pedometer but without changing any of your habits, and note down how many steps you took. For the next two days, aim to increase that figure by 1,000 steps each day. If you feel all right doing that, then increase the figure by a further 1,000 steps for another two days. If you feel good, increase it again. If at any point, however, you become too tired or your legs start to ache, cut back by 500 and stay at that level for three or four days, only increasing the number of steps again when you feel good. Your body will soon get stronger and the activity will get easier.

Using a pedometer

When you first get your pedometer you need to set it up so it measures your step length accurately. Follow the manufacturer's instructions to do this before you start. Make sure your pedometer is firmly fixed – putting it on a very loose waistband will cause it to jiggle about and count extra steps. If you carry your weight on your tummy, the pedometer can tip and it will undercount. Fixing it on the back of your waistband or, in the middle of your bra for women, are alternatives.

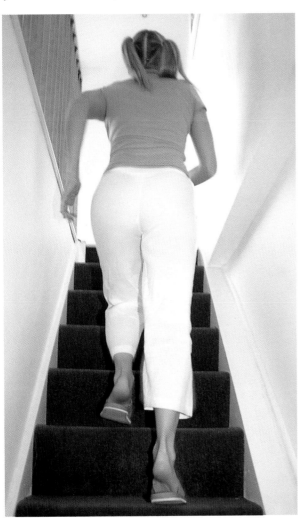

Walk your way thinner

Take every opportunity you can to achieve the daily target of 10,000 steps.

At home

- Pace while you wait for the kettle to boil.
- Walk around during television commercial breaks.
- Pace up and down while you use the phone.
- Unload the grocery shopping one item at a time.
- Never use a remote control.
- Walk around as fast as you can with the vacuum cleaner.
- Walk any journey that is less than a 2-minute car drive.

At work

- Get off the bus one stop before your destination.
- Pace around while you wait for your computer to warm up.
- Use the bathroom on the floor above or below the one on which you work.
- Walk up the stairs instead of taking the lift.
- Deliver messages in person instead of emailing.
- Take the long route around to the sandwich bar or canteen.
- Take a 1-minute walk break between tasks.

Out and about

- Park in the furthest car park space from the shops.
- Walk around the playground while you watch the kids.
- Take the stairs rather than the escalator.
- Walk around the shopping mall once before you start shopping.
- Never go for a 'drive through'.
- Pace up and down while you are waiting for a bus or train.

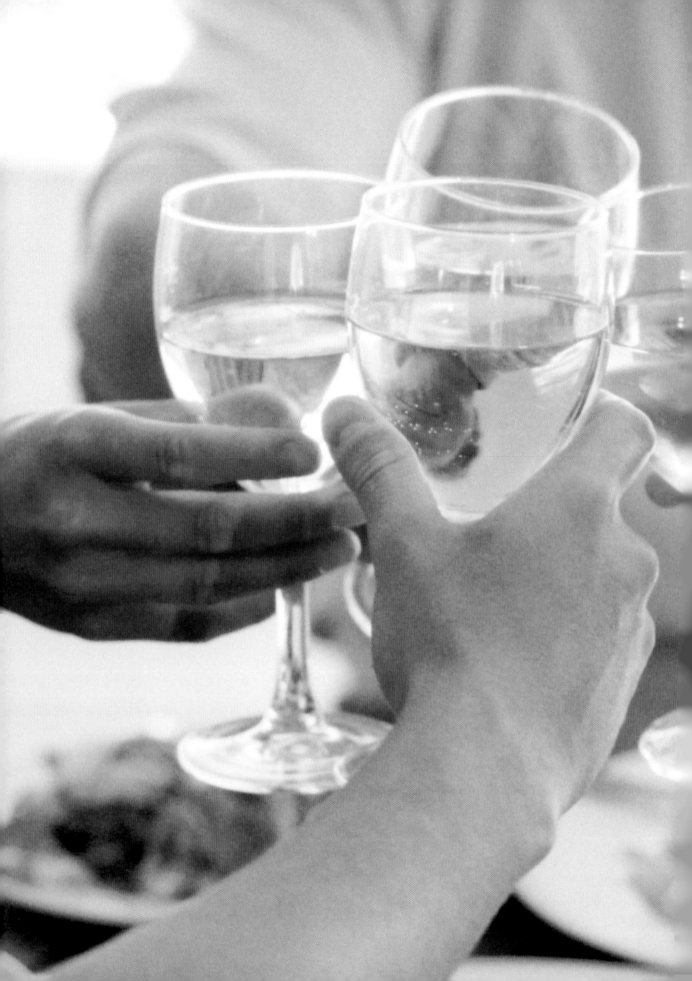

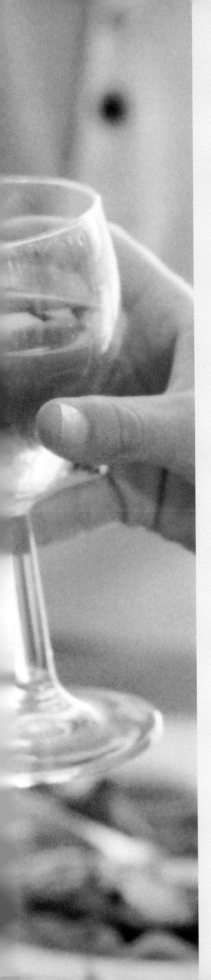

the weekend

So you've reached the weekend. Monday to Friday are done – and so therefore is the portion of your week when you're actively trying to lose weight. All you're trying to do on Saturday and Sunday is maintain your weekday losses. This means the structured plan has gone for two days, you can relax, enjoy nights out with friends, savour a good glass of wine, or take a break from cooking with a takeout – and do it all without guilt.

There are, however, a few simple rules to follow to make sure that your weekend indulgences don't completely cancel out all your hard work during the week. Not only are these 'rules' good ways to maintain your weight over the weekend, they'll also help you keep the weight off when it's gone. In fact, they are the ultimate key to the new slim you.

Rule 1: Eat only to feed your stomach

Every day, 40 per cent of us reach for a food not out of physical hunger, but to feed some other need. You might be filling time because you're bored, trying to cheer yourself up, using sugar to energize you, or even eating because you always eat that food on Saturday night! The end result is you eat calories you don't need and the excess shows on the scales.

Brain food

At weekends it's a good plan, metabolically, to try to continue with your weekday format of three small meals and two small snacks each day. If you find

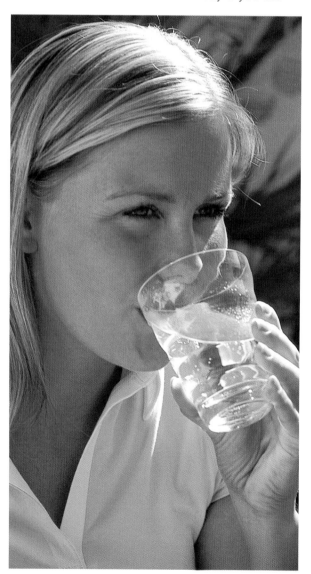

that your three meals are twice the size of your weekday ones and those two snacks turn into nibbling throughout the day, it's not actually your stomach that's making you hungry, it's your brain. Learning when a 'hunger pang' is emotional rather than physical is an important weight control tactic.

Know your enemy

Traditionally, dieters were advised to eat only every 4–5 hours and get used to the actual physical sensations of emptiness, tummy growling and possible lightheadedness that they felt. The trouble with this advice is that when you do eat, you're usually so hungry that you binge. Furthermore, it really doesn't sit well with the little-and-often metabolic-boosting approach you've been taking all week. A better tactic is to use some psychological tricks to identify your needs. Next time you get an urge to eat, ask yourself the following five questions:

❶ Am I craving one particular food right now, or would my hunger actually be satisfied with an apple or carrot sticks?

Why it matters: Emotional hunger is generally linked to a specific food – usually one that's salty, sugary or fatty as these foods create chemicals in the brain that make us feel happier, energized or more relaxed.

What to do: Instead of reaching for the food, try to identify the emotion that wants satisfying and tackle it in a non-food way. Many of the motivation and reward tips on the diet pages can help you do this, but also read up on approaches like aromatherapy or herbal remedies that can help change your mood.

❷ Have I drunk a glass of water in the last hour?

Why it matters: Many of us actually confuse thirst with hunger.

What to do: If you haven't had a drink, then drink a glass of water slowly. If you're still hungry after 15 minutes, then it's OK to eat.

❸ How fast did this hunger come on?

Why it matters: Physical hunger is a gradual process whereas emotional cravings hit like a bolt from the blue. If you're suddenly fixated with eating, it's not your tummy talking, it's your brain.

What to do: Do anything that takes your mind off it – it takes only 10 minutes for this type of craving to pass, so if you can occupy yourself, you won't eat.

❹ If I ate now, could I stop after a few bites, or am I likely to cram it down?

Why it matters: With emotional eating you tend to be on 'autopilot'; sometimes when it's over you're actually shocked at what you've consumed.

What to do: Again, look at what you're really feeling and solve it. Don't have a snack just to settle things down. Once you start eating (even if it's something healthy like carrot sticks) you will keep bingeing until your brain is satisfied – and that could be several hundred 'healthy' calories later.

❺ If I ate now, would I feel satiated and fine when I have finished, or guilty and miserable?

Why it matters: The irony of an emotional eating binge is that when it ends you actually feel worse.

What to do: Remind yourself of that fact. When researchers at Case Western Reserve University in the US asked comfort eaters to tell themselves that the food didn't really make them feel any better, they didn't reach for it.

Real hunger

If, once you've asked yourself all five questions above, you determine that the sensation you are feeling is not an emotional craving but real hunger, then eat – but before you reach for the fridge, remember Rule 2 (see page 106).

Don't weigh yourself at weekends

From Monday to Friday your diet is very low in salt, high in fibre and extremely high in water, so the amount of fluid and waste your body retains is extremely low. At weekends, however, your diet probably includes food higher in salt and carbohydrates, perhaps alcohol and less water/green tea. The result is that you retain fluid and possibly other waste matter, which can add up to (2.2 kg) 5 lb on the scales come Sunday, Monday, or even Tuesday morning. Seeing that is incredibly demotivating, so try to stay off the scales until ideally Friday morning (see page 50).

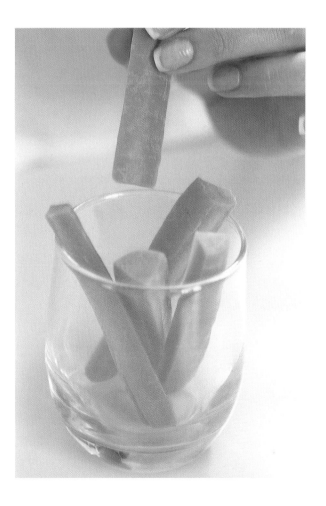

Rule 2: Eat moderate portions

Overeating is often due to overlarge portion sizes and because we don't stop eating when we've had enough. As babies we naturally regulate our food intake this way, but by adulthood we tend to ignore the body's signals that we've had enough. Start listening to them again and discover how this can give you back control around 'danger' foods like chocolate, potato crisps and confectionery.

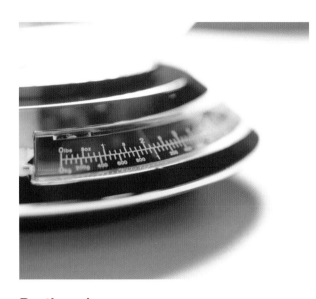

Portion sizes

In the last few years portion sizes across the western world have increased dramatically. According to researchers at New York University, a restaurant serving of steak and the seemingly healthy bagel have both doubled in size. Similarly, in Australia, doctors at the University of Sydney measured 58 different snack foods and found that 86 per cent of them had increased in size in the last ten years alone – half of them having doubled. In the UK, standard 25 g (1 oz) packets of potato crisps are being overtaken by 55 g (2¼ oz) bags, and super-size chocolate bars are rapidly becoming the norm. The result is that many of us now have no idea what a sensible portion of a food actually looks like – and our calorie intake is increasing because of it. Controlling portion sizes is therefore one of the most important things you can to do to tackle weight gain (see box, opposite) – and it's an essential part of enjoying the foods you want to eat at the weekend without gaining weight.

Stop when you're full

While the portion rule is easy to remember, it doesn't always work. When everyday foods are combined in a meal, eating 2–3 moderate portions might still be more than your body needs. Similarly, if you're eating more than one course, the portions of each individual item may be small but together it's a food fest. And with treat foods, psychological factors make it hard to control yourself when you start eating them. When this happens, tapping back into your body's natural signals of satiety (or fullness) will help you get things back under control.

Dealing with treat foods

If you're eating foods like chocolate, biscuits and potato crisps, left to its own devices the body is actually quite good at regulating its calorie intake. It knows whether foods are highly sugary or fatty soon after you start eating them, and actually sends your brain signals that switch off your desire to eat them. You just have to learn to detect these signals.

Try it now with a piece of chocolate – instead of gobbling it down, really savour the flavour. Isn't it incredible? Now chew it for a little, still focusing on that flavour, then swallow. Take another piece and again focus on the flavour. It's probably not that strong now and that incredible mouthwatering sensation has disappeared. A third piece actually tastes kind of ordinary, and a fourth may well taste like chalk. This happens with pretty much every 'treat' food that you eat and it's basically your body's signal that you've had enough.

From now on, listen to that signal. At weekends, whenever you eat those foods you normally feel slightly out of control around, eat them slowly. Savour

Sensible portions of food

Food type	Weight	Portion size
Bagel	100 g (3½ oz)	The size of half a tennis ball
Biscuit	15 g (½ oz)	Similar to the diameter of an electric plug and about 5 mm (¼ in) deep
Bread	40 g (1½ oz)	A slice about the thickness of a pencil
Butter	15 g (½ oz)	The size of a die
Cereal or nuts	25 g (1 oz)	Would fit into the palm of a cupped hand
Cheese	25 g (1 oz)	The size of a matchbox
Chips	100 g (3½ oz)	About 16 standard chips
Chocolate	25 g (1 oz)	Four squares or a matchbox-sized block
Fish fillet	100 g (3½ oz)	About the length and width of a chequebook
Fruit juice	150 ml (¼ pint)	About three fingers deep in a standard tumbler
Meat or poultry	75 g (3 oz)	About the same size and thickness as a deck of cards
Pasta, rice, couscous	50 g (2 oz) dry weight	Roughly 4 tablespoons when cooked
Potato crisps	25 g (1 oz)	About 13 standard potato crisps
Potato, baked	200 g (7 oz)	The size of a tennis ball
Ready-made meal like curry or sweet and sour pork	300 g (10 oz)	A serving would fill a small bowl, about the width of a CD and roughly 5 cm (2½ in) deep
Wine	125 ml (4 fl oz)	About four fingers deep in a small wine glass

every single mouthful and when the pleasure stops, recognize it as your cue to stop eating it.

Foods other than 'treats'

The mechanism above works best with any fatty or sugary food eaten alone. When food tastes are mixed up – as in a meal – it's better to use stomach signals to help prevent you overeating.

Firstly, before every meal, remind yourself of everything you've already eaten today. According to research from the University of Birmingham in the UK, people who do so eat about 50 per cent less at their next meal, possibly because their brain is more primed to deliver satiety signals.

Then, when you do start eating, take your time. It takes 20 minutes for the signals of fullness from your stomach to reach your brain, so chew each mouthful well, put your cutlery down between bites and 'listen' to your body. Watch out for a lack of emptiness in the stomach, a dimming in the smell or taste of food and a slowdown in the speed that you naturally want to eat. Realistically, you will recognize them when they hit. They do so at every meal but are often ignored because we don't want to waste food or because we're used to eating a certain amount. From now on, however, as soon as these feelings occur, stop eating. The worst that can happen is that you stop before you're full and you feel hungry an hour or so later – at which point it's OK to eat.

Rule 3: Make 'healthy' choices

Making healthy choices might sound as if chips and chocolate are suddenly banned on this diet, but that's not true. Controlling weight is simply a matter of balance: if you regulate your calories so that treats and indulgences are balanced with healthier eating choices, you really can have your cake and lose weight, too. There are five main steps to doing this...

❶ Decide on your focal point

When we hear the word 'curry' we tend to think also about rice; say 'cheese' and we think of crackers; mention bacon and we fancy some eggs. However, when it comes to enjoying our food at the weekend, but still cutting down on calories, these food combinations are not always the best choice for our waistlines.

When you eat any meal there's normally a focal point to it, something you're really looking forward to, and everything else just comes along for the ride. For example, what is it about that curry and rice meal you truly enjoy – the spicy richness of the curry or the bland taste of the rice? The chances are that it's the former – so why exactly are you eating the latter? Similarly, if what you're really craving first thing in the morning is bacon, why are you surrounding it with eggs?

On this diet, therefore, before you reach for any individual item in a meal or snack you're going to ask yourself the following question:

On a scale of one to ten, how much do I want this particular food right now?

If your answer is over eight, go for it, serve yourself that food and really enjoy it. If your answer is between six and eight then it's OK to have that food, but serve yourself only about half as much as you think you're going to need, and after each mouthful ask yourself whether you've had enough yet. When the answer to this is 'yes', stop eating it. If your answer to the question scores less than six, then skip that food completely. Sometimes you'll start out planning a big treat, but then realize that chicken and salad actually sounds better now you've thought about it.

❷ Surround your focal point with healthy additions

Again, there are exceptions to every rule in life and the exception to the rule above is fruit and vegetables. It doesn't matter whether they scored a zero on your 'how much do I want these today' question above, you cut them out at your peril. The reason for this is that the average person's body needs about 1.5 kg (3 lb) of food a day, and around 59 nutrients to feel satisfied each day. If it doesn't get these, it will actually start to trigger food cravings to try and fulfil its needs. Fruit and vegetables, however, provide high levels of nutrients and lots of bulk for not many calories – satisfying both your nutritional needs and your desire to lose weight. Because of this, make it a weekend rule always to accompany your 'focal point' food at each meal or snack with at least one piece of fruit or one portion of vegetables – aiming for at least two pieces of fruit and three portions of vegetables each day (see box on page 111).

❸ Check each meal for 'sneaky' calories

Calories come in a number of different disguises. A simple tomato pasta sauce, for example, can contain just 20 calories (84 kJ) per tablespoon, or as many as 250 (1,046 kJ), depending on whether the chef has added oil, cream or butter alongside the primary ingredients. Much of the time, however, these 'sneaky' calories really don't add all that much to your enjoyment of an item, and can be removed, or at least halved, probably without you even noticing.

Watching for 'sneaky' calories in all the foods you choose to eat at the weekend is therefore another way to ensure that the calories you do consume are those you are enjoying eating.

Avoiding 'sneaky' calories

Use a spray oil when cooking. Replacing 1 tablespoon oil or 25 g (1 oz) butter with a few sprays of oil to fry ingredients like onions or garlic will cut 100 calories (418 kJ) from a recipe. Either buy one at the supermarket or make up your own in a plastic spray bottle, using ⅓ olive oil to ⅔ water.

- Pat the fat. Using kitchen roll to absorb surface oil from fatty foods cuts calories – for example, 45 calories (188 kJ) from a slice of pizza and 30–40 calories (126–167 kJ) from a burger or sausage.
- Chilling foods like soups or stews after cooking, then scraping off the layer of fat that forms on the surface will cut about 100 calories (418 kJ) per dish. You can also do this with canned goods like chilli if you chill them before you open the can.
- Cut all obvious fat from meats and remove skin from poultry. Also buy lean cuts of potentially fatty meats like beef instead of marbled cuts.
- If cooking with mince, dry fry it then, once browned, tip the mince into a sieve. Pour boiling water over the meat to rinse off any excess fat. Shake well, and then add it to your recipe.

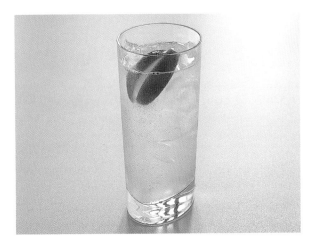

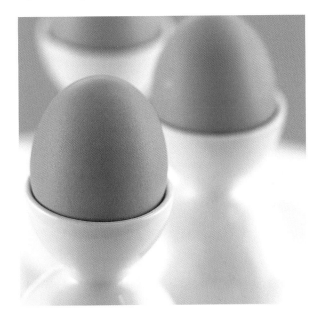

- If a recipe calls for more than 1 whole egg, you can replace half of them with just egg whites – these contain 15 calories (63 kJ), while a whole egg is about 90 (377 kJ).
- If you want to fry chips, cut them large as the more surface area an item has, the less fat it absorbs. Also, fry them in small portions rather than putting lots in at once, which cools the oil and increases the time for which they need to be in it.
- Dilute drinks. Orange juice or wine diluted with soda water halves the calories. In addition, don't drink calories if you don't have to. A vodka tonic with real tonic contains 150 calories (628 kJ), a vodka tonic with slimline tonic contains just 50 (209 kJ).
- Watch out for the calories in condiments. The average person consumes 3,000 calories (12,552 kJ) of ketchup, mayonnaise, salad cream and other condiments a month! Swap full-fat versions for low-calories ones, or – even better – replace them with virtually zero-calorie condiments like hot sauce, balsamic vinegar, mustard and lemon juice.

❹ Beware eating amnesia

The average dieter not following an organized plan underestimates the amount of calories they consume each day by at least 400 calories (1,674 kJ). 'Forgotten' calories are the reason – those potato crisps you ate out of your partner's packet, the piece of cheese you had while standing by the fridge, and the leftovers from the children's dinner you nibbled instead of throwing away. Be very, very careful of 'forgotten' calories at the weekend as they can destroy everything. Here are some ways to avoid them:

- Make it a weekend rule to eat only as part of one of your three meals or two snacks each day.
- Never eat standing up, or even at any place other than the table.
- Always serve food on a plate or other piece of crockery – after all, how can you tell what you're eating if you don't see it laid out in front of you?
- Be very conscious of portion sizes if you're serving from large packets, or into large containers. Researchers at the University of Illinois in the US found that people eat up to 50 per cent more of snack foods when they are eaten from a large packet and they pour 76 per cent more orange juice into a large wide glass than a tall thin one. Remember, portion control is everything.

❹ Eating out at the weekend

For many of us, eating out or getting a takeout is a big part of our weekend food consumption. It's not necessarily a bad thing, but remember this one fact: the person who eats out three times a week consumes one-third more calories each week than someone who eats out only once. The reason is that when we eat out, or have a takeout meal, portion sizes are normally considerably larger than we would serve ourselves at home and it's impossible to tell how many calories are in a restaurant dish unless you're standing over the chef while it's being made. On most diets, therefore, you're advised to avoid eating out entirely while trying to lose weight. On this diet that's not necessary – you can eat out and still maintain your weight if you use one of the two approaches described opposite.

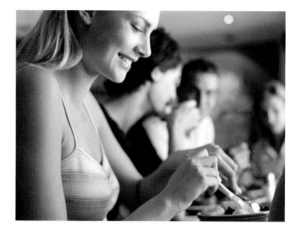

Restaurant terms

If you're at a formal restaurant, the menu is likely to include some culinary terms you may be unsure of. In these cases it's good to know which food descriptions should get the green light, and which to steer clear of:

Green light choices
- **Au jus:** in its own juices
- **Brochette:** skewered like a kebab
- **Broiled:** cooked in water or wine
- **Carpaccio:** thin raw slices of meat or fish
- **Consommé:** a thin broth soup
- **Grilled:** as you'd expect
- **Steamed:** another good choice as no oil is used in steaming
- **Stir-fried:** similarly, very little oil is used in stir-frying
- **Tartare:** chopped raw meat or fish, flavoured with herbs

Foods to steer clear of
- **Aioli:** garlic mayonnaise
- **'Aise':** sauces ending in this tend to be high in fat
- **Au beurre:** cooked in butter
- **Au gratin:** cooked with cheese
- **Breaded or battered:** also often fried
- **Confit:** cooked in its own fat
- **Crispy:** normally means fried
- **En croûte:** cooked in pastry
- **Sautéed:** cooked in butter

Approach 1

Before you go out, read again the weekend rules outlined on the previous pages and use the tactics to help you regulate what you're eating. Particular things to avoid are: ordering courses you're not really hungry for just because you're 'out for dinner', consuming 'wasted' calories in things like full-fat dressing poured over your salad (have it served on the side, or ask for a plain balsamic dressing instead), eating huge portions of foods just because you've been served them, and eating things you're not really enjoying because they happen to have been served with your dish. Think about how each rule applies to restaurant eating and aim to keep things under control naturally.

Approach 2

The second tactic when eating out is to order the healthiest options on the menu from the outset (see box opposite). While calories will vary, some dishes are generally more healthy than others, so learn to recognize the best dishes to order.

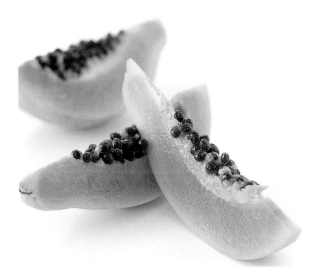

What if you hate fruit and vegetables?

If you believe you don't like fruit and vegetables you probably haven't experimented enough with the loads of different types out there, or with ways of serving them. Try the tips below to help find things that please your palate:

- Exotic fruits like mango, papaya, star fruit and guava have sweeter, more subtle tastes than traditional fruits like apples or citrus. If you haven't tried them, then do.
- Alter the taste of bitter vegetables like spinach, cabbage, cauliflower or kale by sprinkling them with lemon juice.
- Many people who don't like boiled vegetables when served enjoy the taste of them raw or lightly steamed.
- Conversely, some fruits taste preferable to when cooked. Try baked apples, poached pears, or grilled pineapple or mango.

- Don't assume that if you didn't like a vegetable as a child, you won't like it now. As children we have more tastebuds than when we become adults, which makes flavours more intense. When taste dulls with age, strong foods like olives or Brussels sprouts actually taste better.
- Most people do like the taste of sweet or creamy fruit and vegetables like carrots, corn, peas, avocados, strawberries and bananas, so if all else fails, stick with these.

Ordering wisely

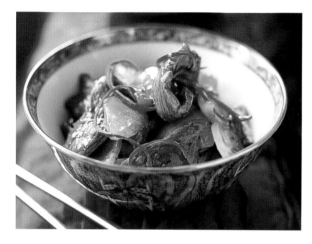

At the Italian restaurant
STARTERS
- Minestrone or a non-creamy tomato soup
- Parma ham with melon or figs
- Vegetable starters like asparagus with Parmesan

MAINS
- Pasta with tomato/vegetable sauces
- Pasta with seafood sauce
- Stuffed peppers
- Thin-crust vegetarian pizzas

DESSERTS
- Sorbet and granita

At the Chinese/Japanese restaurant
STARTERS
- Chicken and sweetcorn soup
- Hot and sour soup
- Sashimi
- Sushi rolls

MAINS
- Any dish in black bean sauce
- Any dish in oyster sauce
- Any stir-fry or dish described as 'with vegetables'
- Bento boxes (mixed lunchboxes containing sushi, sashimi, miso soup, pickled vegetables, etc. – but leave out the tempura)
- Steamed dumplings
- Chop suey
- Plain rice

DESSERTS
- Green tea ice cream
- Lychees (fresh, or canned in natural juice, not syrup)

At the Thai restaurant
STARTERS
- Tom yum soup
- Thai fishcakes

MAINS
- Stir-fries with chilli/ginger/basil/lemon grass (no coconut cream)
- Pad thai noodles (go easy on the peanuts)
- Thai salads (with chilli/vinegar dressing – not coconut cream)

DESSERTS
- Fresh fruit

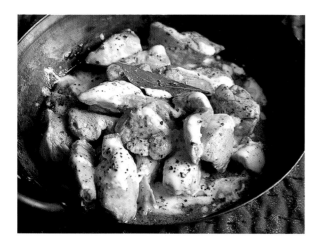

At the Indian restaurant
STARTERS
- Small portion of chicken tikka or tandoori chicken
- Poppadums with yogurt dip

MAINS
- Chicken tikka or tandoori chicken (if you haven't already had this as a starter)
- Vegetables or seafood in tomato- or yogurt-based sauces
- Plain rice

DESSERTS
- Fresh fruit
- Small portion of kulfi

At the Mexican restaurant
STARTERS
- Black bean soup
- Tortilla chips with salsa (restrict yourself to about 25 chips)

MAINS
- Fajitas (go easy on the soured cream)
- Plain bean or chicken burritos (no cheese or soured cream)
- Vegetarian chilli

DESSERTS
- Best avoided

At the steakhouse
STARTERS
- Prawn cocktail
- Melon
- Minestrone soup

MAINS
- Lean steak with salad or baked potato
- Plain fish fillet with salad or baked potato
- Grilled gammon with pineapple and salad or baked potato
- Roasted chicken with vegetables

DESSERTS
- Fruit salad
- Small portion of ice cream

Fast food or café food
- Small plain hamburger
- Chicken burgers made with unbreaded chicken
- Plain salad with low-calorie dressing
- Small fries
- Baked potato with baked beans (no butter or margarine) or cottage cheese
- Sandwiches made with lean ham, chicken or roast beef and salad (no butter or margarine)

Temptation action plan

The point of the Temptation Action Plan is to get you through those weekends when your willpower just seems to have gone on holiday. For some women this occurs prior to the beginning of their menstrual cycle, for other people it might be triggered by special occasions or, most frustratingly, for no obvious reason at all. When those days hit, here are the tricks to get you back on track.

When eating out...

- Order first. We eat 44 per cent more food when we eat with others than when we eat alone – possibly because it's very easy for our good intentions to get shortcircuited by a dining companion ordering a starter, a main course and the extra bread basket.
- If you still don't think you can trust yourself, tell a friend what you would like to order, then go to the bathroom until the waiter has gone so no one can change your mind.
- Never drink more than one alcoholic drink before a meal. Every drink you have affects a different part of your body or brain – but it takes only two drinks for the inhibitory part of your brain to be affected, making it much harder to make good food choices.

- If you decide you're full and everyone else is still eating, put your napkin over the food so you can no longer see it, or signal to the waiter to take the plate away. If you feel it's rude to do either of these while your companions are still eating, either put the handles of your cutlery into the food itself, or pour salt over the leftovers so you won't pick any more.
- At a buffet, remember the 'six out of ten' rule (see page 108) – any food that scores less than that on your 'I want it' scale gets left on the table and its place taken by fruit or vegetable accompaniments.
- Split desserts with others – you tend to be too embarrassed to eat more than your fair share if you do this.
- Avoid facing the buffet table at parties or sitting close to the peanut bowl in a bar – people eat twice as much of an item if it's within their field of vision than if it's out of sight.

When at home...

- For the same reason as above, don't store treat foods where you can see them.
- Write down everything you eat at the weekend before you do so – and put this list somewhere noticeable like the fridge or pantry door. Sometimes the act of writing it down can make you reach for a healthier choice, or put the item back in the fridge completely. If you're more of a visual person, photographing everything with a digital camera can also work.
- Set yourself a night-time curfew – don't allow yourself to eat anything after your evening meal, or after 8pm or whatever time you set yourself. If you have to, put a chair in front of the fridge so you have to think before you open it.

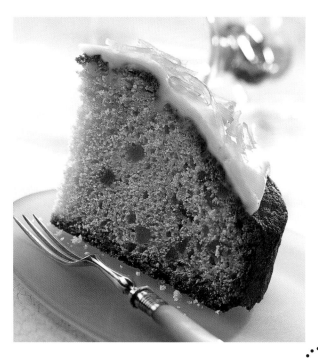

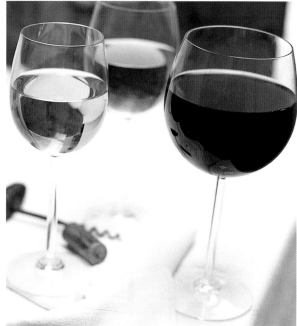

- Chew gum (a low-sugar or sugar-free variety). It stops you putting food in your mouth without thinking – and as an added bonus, for every 1 hour you chew you burn up as much as 11 calories (46 kJ)!
- Ask other people to clear away the leftovers when you have finished eating. It'll stop you eating that final slice of cake instead of throwing it away or wrapping it in cling film.
- When you're putting leftovers away in the fridge, ensure that they are in sealed containers with lids on. Not only will it help keep food fresher, the extra few seconds it takes to remove the lid (especially if it's a slightly tight lid that you have to fight with) can be enough in itself to prevent mindless nibbling.

Don't despair

Always remember, if you do overeat completely at one meal, don't beat yourself up over it. That meal will not destroy your entire diet, only what you do next can do that. Let that meal go, and at the next meal really focus on what your body (not your brain) is telling you it wants – the chances are that it will be something light and healthy and you'll feel fuller faster than normal. Remember that your body naturally balances out what it needs each day if only you listen to it.

Female friendly tips

If you find that cravings strike just before your period, then it might help to take a magnesium supplement. It'll also be important for you to eat little and often – a lot of pre-menstrual food cravings occur because blood sugar is even more sensitive at this time.

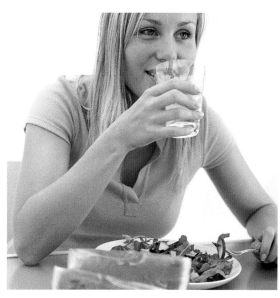

Rule 4: Move your body

While Rules 1 to 3 should ensure you don't eat more calories than you're using up each weekend, following this final rule makes it 100 per cent certain. You've already introduced exercise into your weekly life (and keeping up those 10,000 steps each day is recommended at weekends, too), but a little extra activity as well will help ensure you maintain your weight while eating your weekend treats.

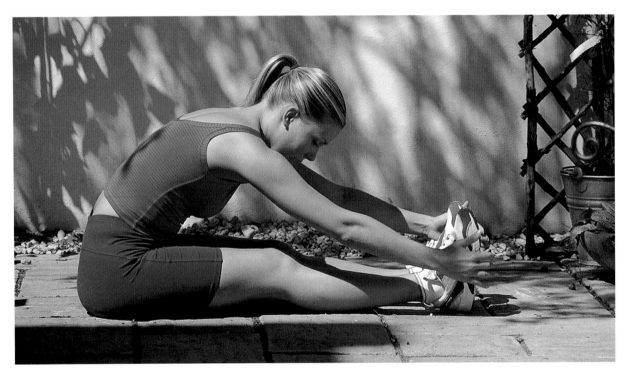

Think of exercise as fun

As a child you ran, cycled and skipped and it was fun; when you were a teenager, you danced the night away and/or played in sports teams, and again it was fun. In adulthood, though, most of us stop seeing exercise as fun and regard it as a chore, something that must hurt and must take place in the gym. The truth, however, is that any kind of activity can burn calories, and help you maintain your weight. And if you can do at least 30 minutes of fun activity each day at the weekend (or one 60-minute session), you will boost results. This could involve that big spring cleaning job you're itching to tackle, doing some decorating, just walking to the shops instead of driving, or something more sporty like one of the ideas here.

AEROBICS

Burns **210–400 calories (879–1,674 kJ)** per 30 minutes (depending on class)
It's for you if: You like exercising with others and you have good coordination.
Top tip: Choose the class that fits your level – low-impact aerobics is good for beginners.

AQUA AEROBICS

Burns **200 calories (837 kJ)** per 30 minutes
It's for you if: You like exercising with others, but lack coordination or fitness (the water hides both).
Top tip: The deeper the water, the harder you'll work as resistance is greater. If you're a beginner, start in water no deeper than your chest.

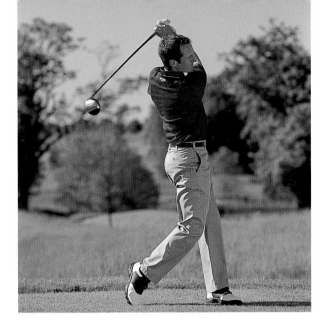

BADMINTON
Burns **275 calories (1,151 kJ)** per 30 minutes
It's for you if: You'd love to play tennis, but can't hit a ball – the shuttlecock is easier to follow.
Top tip: Start with a plastic shuttlecock, which is more likely to go where it's supposed to.

CYCLING
Burns **300 calories (1,255 kJ)** per 30 minutes
It's for you if: You like scenery while you exercise or you're injury prone (there's no impact).
Top tip: If your bottom aches while you cycle, raise yourself out of the saddle periodically to release the lactic acid that builds up and makes you ache.

DANCING
Burns **200 calories (837 kJ)** per 30 minutes for ballroom, **350 calories (1,464 kJ)** for fast disco
It's for you if: Exercise has to be fun.
Top tip: If you can't fit in nights out, dance at home – just put on a favourite CD and enjoy.

DOG WALKING
Burns **150 calories (628 kJ)** per 30 minutes
It's for you if: You aren't that fit yet.
Top tip: You'll go further if you keep the dog on a fixed-length lead rather than an extending one.

FRISBEE
Burns **100 calories (418 kJ)** per 30 minutes
It's for you if: You can catch, you like to be outside, or you want to play with the children.
Top tip: Control your Frisbee throwing by flicking from your wrist, not your elbow.

GARDENING
Burns **150 calories (628 kJ)** per 30 minutes
It's for you if: You like nurturing things and you don't want exercise to feel like exercise.
Top tip: To boost calorie burning, focus on the more intensive tasks like weeding, lawn mowing and potting.

GOLF
Burns **122 calories (510 kJ)** per 30 minutes (carrying your own clubs)
It's for you if: You like competition, but not team sports or anything too vigorous.
Top tip: On your initial swing, really aim to drive through the ball not just hit it.

HIKING
Burns **150 calories (628 kJ)** per 30 minutes
It's for you if: You're on a budget, you like the outdoors and don't mind exercising alone.
Top tip: Wear proper hiking boots – trainers don't always provide enough ankle support on uneven ground.

HORSERIDING
Burns **134 calories (561 kJ)** per 30 minutes
It's for you if: You're not scared of horses or heights, and you like speed.
Top tip: Take lessons – if you're fairly fit and confident you can be trotting in 2 hours.

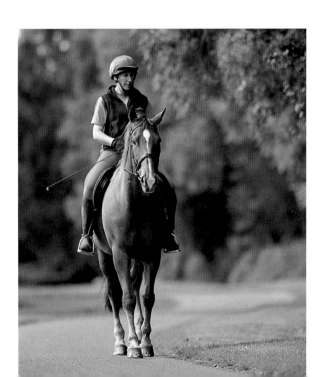

IN-LINE OR ICE SKATING

Burns **193 calories (808 kJ)** per 30 minutes

It's for you if: You can balance, you want to exercise with the children, or you like exercise to feel fun.

Top tip: Keep your knees bent as you skate – stiffening up alters your balance. Outstretched arms help, too.

INDOOR ROCK CLIMBING

Burns **349 calories (1,460 kJ)** per 30 minutes

It's for you if: You're not scared of heights and you like to exercise alone.

Top tip: Push yourself up with your leg muscles – pulling with your arms is too tiring.

JOGGING

Burns **300 calories (1,255 kJ)** per 30 minutes

It's for you if: You like competing against yourself, don't mind exercising alone and are on a budget.

Top tip: Try to run with your whole foot, landing on your heels and rolling up through your toes.

KAYAKING

Burns **190 calories (795 kJ)** per 30 minutes

It's for you if: You live near water and enjoy scenery while you work out.

Top tip: Don't power the paddle by pulling it back with the hand closest to the water. Instead, push forwards with the arm closest to your body – it's less tiring.

MARTIAL ARTS

Burns **160 calories (669 kJ)** per 30 minutes

It's for you if: You enjoy mentally absorbing hobbies.

Top tip: Martial arts depend on focus so arrive for classes 10 minutes early to help you relax.

PILATES

Burns **150 calories (628 kJ)** per 30 minutes

It's for you if: You want a low-impact exercise – and would also like to improve your posture or achieve a flat tummy.

Top tip: Take at least one class before trying a video or book at home. If you don't get in the right positions the exercises don't work – and it's hard to know that without expert help.

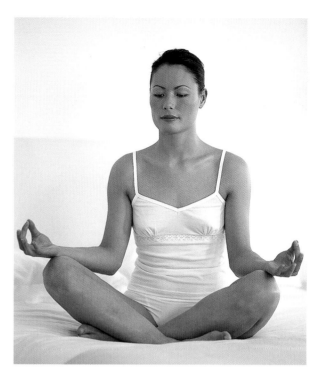

PLAYGROUND FUN

(playing with the kids on the swings, monkey bars etc.)

Burns **200 calories (837 kJ)** per 30 minutes

It's for you if: You have children and you're on a tight budget.

Top tip: Go when the playground is quiet and really enjoy yourselves.

ROPE SKIPPING

Burns **300 calories (1,255 kJ)** per 30 minutes

It's for you if: You're already quite fit and you want a workout you can do at home.

Top tip: Your rope needs to be long enough to turn easily, but not too loose. To test it, stand in position, standing on the rope. Pull it tight, then release it about 8 cm (3 in).

SKIING

Burns **220 calories (920 kJ)** per 30 minutes

It's for you if: You have good balance and you like speed.

Top tip: Remember, you don't need to ski outside. Many big towns have indoor slopes.

SOCCER

Burns **220 calories (920 kJ)** per 30 minutes

It's for you if: You like team sports and/or you have children.

Top tip: To get the ball to go where you want, hit it in the centre, pushing it towards the direction in which you wish it to move.

SQUASH

Burns **310 calories (1,297 kJ)** per 30 minutes

It's for you if: You're competitive, you're fairly fit already and you like fast-paced exercise.

Top tip: Always keep your eye on the ball – most people look at the wall in front of them instead.

SWIMMING

Burns **200–300 calories (837–1,255 kJ)** per 30 minutes (depending on stroke)

It's for you if: You like exercising alone, you're injury prone (there's no impact) and you like water.

Top tip: Buy goggles – even if you don't put your head under the water they help you keep going for longer, burning more calories.

TABLE TENNIS

Burns **126 calories (527 kJ)** per 30 minutes

It's for you if: You want to play with your children or you want exercise that's fun.

Top tip: Keep the ball low on the table and aim to hit it with the middle of the paddle.

TEN PIN BOWLING

Burns **150 calories (628 kJ)** per 30 minutes

It's for you if: You want exercise to be social and you're not hugely fit.

Top tip: Ask the alley to put the sides up for you – it stops the ball going down the gulley and makes it more fun for beginners and children.

YOGA

Burns **100–200 calories (418–837 kJ)** per 30 minutes (depending on type)

It's for you if: You don't want a high-impact workout and you'd like to de-stress too.

Top tip: If you're finding it hard to get into certain stretches, having something to push against (like a neck tie) can help gently extend things.

Top 5 excuses dismissed

I don't have time

Exercise in the morning – getting up 30 minutes earlier gives you all the time you need. Or, split your workouts into three 10-minute bursts, which is actually better for your metabolism.

I'm not fit enough to exercise

Then start off with walking, trying to stay out for longer and longer each time. When you reach a point when you can walk for 20 minutes in one go at a brisk pace, then you can think about other sports.

I'm too big to go to the gym

A lot of people who are overweight believe this, but most gym staff and other exercisers will support you – and if they don't, find a more friendly gym! Or, try home exercise with videos or DVDs, a treadmill or exercise bike.

I have children and can't leave them

Then don't. Childhood obesity is one of the biggest health crises of our time and lack of activity is believed to be the main reason. Do activities that your children can do with you.

I can't afford to exercise

It's a myth that working out needs to be costly. Walking is free, running requires only a supportive pair of trainers, and most leisure centres offer swimming sessions and fitness classes at inexpensive prices.

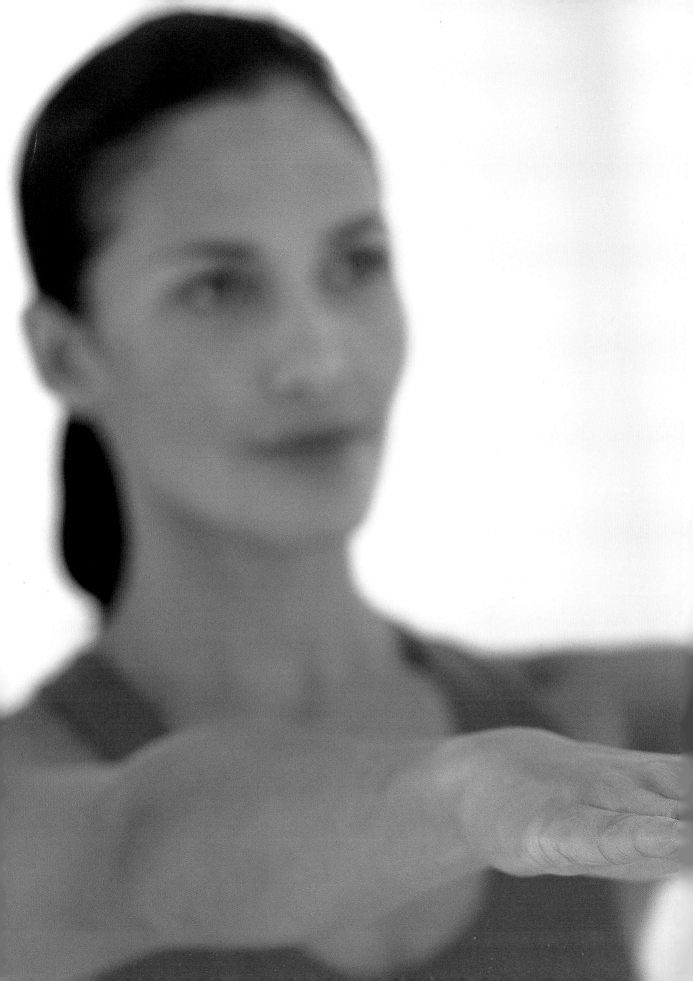

winning the weight-loss war

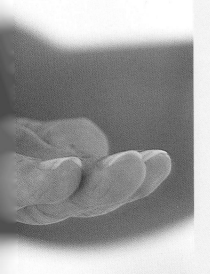

Believe it or not, when it comes to losing weight, those first few weeks and months when you're actively trying to lose your excess weight can actually be the easy part. The real struggle comes in keeping it off.

Many of the tactics you've learnt on both the weekday plan and your weekends off have taught you how to handle yourself around all sorts of foods, not just those with hardly any calories, and this is the number one tip you need to stay slim. But it's not the only tip – read on for some more strategies to help keep you leaner for life. If you're reading these pages before you''ve started on your weight loss journey, then that's great, but the most important day to read them is the day you reach your goal weight, so keep them close at hand.

How to keep the weight off

While keeping off lost weight may be the hardest part of any diet, the actual rules you have to follow to achieve it couldn't be more simple. There are just three main areas you need to master: what and how much you eat; how much you move – consciously and otherwise; and thinking yourself thin.

What to eat

Once your weight has decreased, if you try to go back to eating the same number of calories as before, you'll gain weight. On average, for every 0.5 kg (1 lb) of fat you lose, you have to decrease your daily intake by about 10 calories (42 kJ) to keep your weight stable.

For a more precise measurement, multiply your weight in pounds (to convert kg to lb, simply multiply by 2.2) by one of the following factors:
- By 12 if you have a sedentary job and do no or only gentle exercise,
- By 13 if you have a sedentary job but exercise intensely (i.e. more than walking) for at least 30 minutes most days,
- By 15 if you are very active during the day and/or exercise intensely for at least an hour most days.

The figure you end up with gives you the daily number of calories you can consume without putting on weight. (If you are more familiar with kiloJoules, multiply this figure by 4.2 to convert calories to kiloJoules).

Now you know your recommended daily calorie consumption, *what* you eat is really up to you, but remember that meal skipping slows metabolism and in every study ever done on successful slimmers it's been found that breakfast eaters have an easier time maintaining their weight than those who skip it. It's also been found that those who find it easiest to maintain their weight also consume at least five portions of fruit and vegetables every single day. Since you have only a finite number of calories that you can eat each day before you start to gain weight, it's far better to spend those calories on things you enjoy rather than wasting them. So even

now, switch to low-fat versions of as many foods as you can and avoid those 'sneaky' calories (see page 108).

Lastly, remember it takes about six weeks to break a habit, but a lot less time to make one. On this plan you learned to survive having only truly high-fat and high-calorie foods at the weekends, so why bring them back in during the week now? A good rule to live by is 80 per cent 'healthy' choices, 20 per cent treats – but try to avoid always having those treats at the same time each day, which sets up patterns that can lead to overeating. Keep your diet varied and remember… nothing in moderation will make you fat.

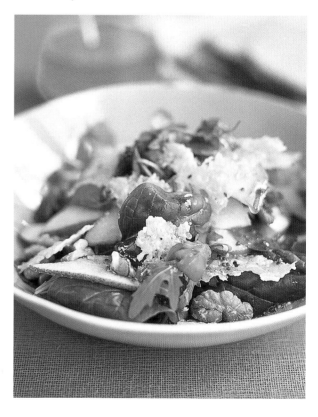

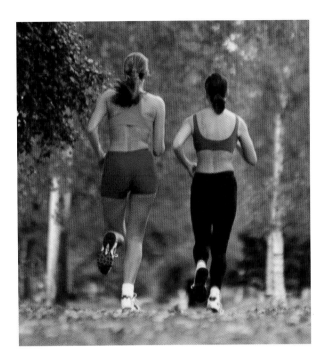

How much to move

The answer here is, as much as possible. When US organization the National Weight Registry tracked people who had lost at least 31 kg (70 lb) and successfully kept it off for more than six years, they found the one thing they had in common was that every single one of them walked, or exercised in some other way, for at least 1 hour a day.

Really try to make the activity that you started during this diet part of your life. Keep up those 10,000 steps a day – maybe even try to increase it to 15,000 or 20,000 some days – and, if you took up new sports or active hobbies at weekends (see page 116), don't let these slide now that you're no longer trying to lose weight. Keep yourself motivated by entering races or charity events involving your new hobby, take lessons to improve your technique or even set up your own ten pin bowling or soccer team. It'll also do you good to add different activities, or shake up your workout by doing it in a different order or at a different pace every now and again – our bodies get used to exercise and after a while you don't get the same effects, so do vary things.

The NEAT factor

It's not just intensive exercise that makes the difference between fat and thin. In 2005 researchers at the Mayo Clinic in the US found that the biggest difference between thin people and those battling with their weight was their NEAT factor. NEAT stands for Non-Exercise Activity Thermogenesis, which accounts for all the calories you burn each day fidgeting (which can apparently wipe out almost 1,000 calories/4,184 kJ a day!), standing up instead of sitting down and waving your arms when you speak. So really try to focus on increasing the amount of this type of movement that you do each day.

Tips for those days when it all seems too tough

Every exerciser has these: you know you should get out there and move, but it just seems too much trouble. Here are some ways to motivate yourself:

- Use the 10 minute rule. Tell yourself all you have to do is go and do your workout for 10 minutes. If you're still not enjoying it after that then you are allowed to go home – the thing is that nine times out of ten, you don't.
- Do some fast bursts. It might sound completely unlike anything you feel like at the moment, but sometimes adding a bit of speed to your exercise plan can give you a burst of adrenaline that re-energizes you. All you have to do is spend 30 seconds every minute or two doing your particular exercise at the fastest pace you can. When 30 seconds is over, slow down for as long as it takes for you to get your breath back, then go again.
- Switch locations. If you normally work out at a gym, try taking your exercise outside for once – go for a walk or jog in the fresh air. If you normally exercise outside, jump in the car and take yourself to somewhere new – the change of scenery will make it feel like a new workout.
- Play some music. Studies at the Human Performance Laboratory at the University of Tennessee have discovered that exercisers find working out more enjoyable if they do it to music. As an added bonus, you may even end up working out for longer than normal when you use this tip. Studies at Springfield College in Massachusetts (which specializes in physical education) have found women work out for 25 per cent longer when they listen to music – and men go 29 per cent further.

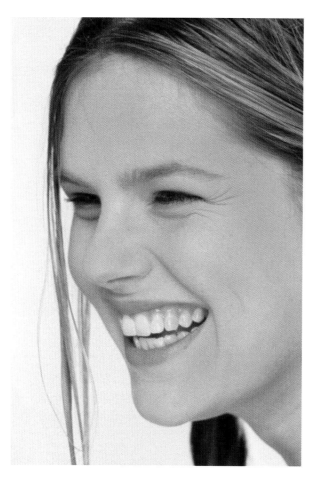

starting with those areas that contributed to your emotional eating urges. Start to look at approaches to help tackle the root cause of those emotions. For example, if you're incredibly stressed at work, look at the reasons why. Is it the systems in place, in which case how can you change them? Is it that you leave things to the last minute, in which case work on tips to tackle procrastination. If you worry about things before they happen, check out self-help books that aim to stop this kind of negative thinking. The more emotional triggers you eliminate from your life, the better your life will be.

Keep portions moderate ... and only eat until full

These two techniques (see page 106) mean that from now on there's no such thing as a bad food in your life, so never forget them.

Eat only the calories you really want

Mindless eating is not only the enemy of the dieter, it's also the enemy of the maintainer. Avoid nibbling out of packets, from other people's plates and just because you're in the kitchen. If you find it tough, start keeping a food diary. It might seem like something you should do only when you're dieting, but that's not true. Writing down your daily food intake can help you spot extra calories creeping in as soon as they start – and before they become a habit you need to break. You don't necessarily have to do it every day – once a week, or for two or three days a month can work just as well.

Have a happy weight band

Weight does fluctuate from day to day, especially if you're a woman at the mercy of hormonal fluctuations. That's why having one goal for your perfect weight isn't the best plan: instead, have a 1–2 kg (2–4 lb) zone in which you aim to stay. Weigh yourself once a week or once a month – if at any point you go over the highest figure on that buffer, make it a rule to cut back calories and increase exercise to get that extra weight off.

Don't feel guilty

Never feel guilty about a big meal, a big day or even a big weekend of eating. Guilt just causes potential emotional eating problems for you to overcome. If you have a few days where every

- Tell yourself you can have a treat afterwards. Research from the Cooper Institute for Aerobics Research in the US has found people are nearly three times more likely to work out if they give themselves a reward for doing it. This does not, however, mean a big chocolate bar. Think of something non-food related like 20 minutes in the gym sauna, an uninterrupted half hour in front of the television or even a day off the housework.

Think thin

If your brain is engaged in losing weight it'll be a lot easier for your body to be involved, too. All the tactics you learnt during your weekends off help you to think thin – and there are a few extra that also come into play when the weight has gone. So remember the following guidelines…

Feed hunger not emotion

Now that your weight-loss project is over, perhaps think about changing other areas of your life, too, sensible eating habit you've learnt goes out of the window, don't worry about it – just get back into your sensible eating habits as soon as you can. Don't, for example, make the mistake of arriving home from holiday on a Wednesday and telling yourself you'll start eating well again on Monday. As soon as you decide enough is enough, get back to eating well at your next meal or even snack.

Beware other people's reactions

While you might be thrilled that you've lost weight, others might not. Friends can be jealous and partners may feel threatened, so watch for sneaky saboteurs trying to give you extra food. Also watch out for over-carers – people asking you whether you should really be eating that food after you've worked so hard. They might think they're helping,

but it can cause you to rebel and actually eat more of the food as you try to show that you know best – and that doesn't always turn out well!

Keep setting yourself goals

Finally, remember the day will come when people will stop noticing that you have lost weight. This doesn't make it any less of an achievement, but it can be the time when your motivation starts to slip. If you need positive reinforcement to help keep you motivated, set yourself a new goal like learning to swim or running a 5 km (3 mile) race. This will keep your weight under control and give you the big mental 'cheers' that you enjoy. Who knows, one day you might find yourself crossing the finishing line of a marathon or even a triathlon! From now on, the only way is up.

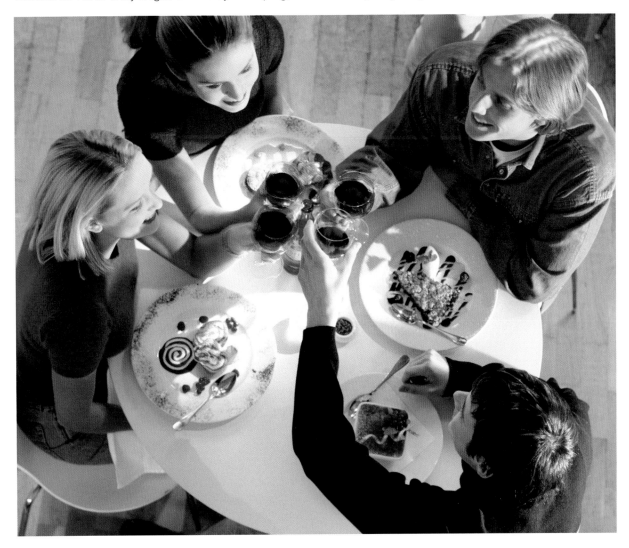

Index

Acknowledgements

Executive Editor: Nicola Hill
Project Editor: Kate Tuckett
Executive Art Editor: Joanna MacGregor
Designer: Ginny Zeal
Senior Production Controller: Ian Paton

Special Photography © Octopus Publishing Group Limited/Russell Sadur.

Other photography:

Corbis UK Ltd/Jutta Klee 10.
Getty Images/Nancy Brown 124; /James Darell 110; /Christian Hoehn 18; /Image Source 106; /Romilly Lockyer 8 bottom; /VCL/Spencer Rowell 125; /Thinkstock 102; /Victoria Yee 7 bottom.
Image Source 17.
Octopus Publishing Group Limited/Bob Atkins 117 bottom; /Clive Bozzard-Hill 49, 55, 61, 69; /Jean Cazals 115 top right; /Stephen Conroy 31 right, 109 top; /Jeremy Hopley 21 top, 109 bottom; /William Lingwood 8 top, 30, 52; /David Loftus 29; /Jason Lowe 113; /Angus Murray 117 top; /Ian O'Leary 25 bottom; /Lis Parsons 3 top, 19, 21 bottom, 25 top, 33, 57, 63, 111; /Mike Prior 23; /Peter Pugh-Cook 11, 28 top, 101, 104, 105, 115 bottom right, 116; /William Reavell 20, 37, 39, 45, 71, 112; /Craig Robertson 122; /Gareth Sambidge 13, 35, 41, 43, 47, 51, 53 left, 59, 65, 67, 73; /Simon Smith 3 bottom, 115 top left; /Ian Wallace 7 top, 31 left, 53 right, 100, 114.
Photodisc 6, 9, 12, 16, 17, 22, 123